An Atlas of Investigation and Management
OBESITY

An Atlas of Investigation and Management

OBESITY

BS Aditya, MRCP
Consultant Physician
Diabetes and Endocrinology Department
University Hospital Aintree
Liverpool, UK

JPH Wilding, DM, FRCP
Professor of Medicine
University of Liverpool
Honorary Consultant Physician
Head of Department of Obesity and Endocrinology
University Hospital Aintree
Liverpool, UK

Foreword by

W Philip T James, CBE, FRSE, MD, DSc
President, International Association for the Study of Obesity (IASO)
Honorary Professor of Nutrition
London School of Hygiene and Tropical Medicine
London, UK

CLINICAL PUBLISHING

OXFORD

Clinical Publishing
an imprint of Atlas Medical Publishing Ltd
Oxford Centre for Innovation
Mill Street, Oxford OX2 0JX, UK

Tel: +44 1865 811116
Fax: +44 1865 251550
Email: info@clinicalpublishing.co.uk
Web: www.clinicalpublishing.co.uk

Distributed in USA and Canada by:
Clinical Publishing
30 Amberwood Parkway
Ashland OH 44805, USA

Tel: 800-247-6553 (toll free within US and Canada)
Fax: 419-281-6883
Email: order@bookmasters.com

Distributed in UK and Rest of World by:
Marston Book Services Ltd
PO Box 269
Abingdon
Oxon OX14 4YN, UK

Tel: +44 1235 465500
Fax: +44 1235 465555
Email: trade.orders@marston.co.uk

ISBN-13   978 1 84692 027 1
ISBN e-book   978 1 84692 619 8

**The publisher makes no representation, express or implied, that the dosages in this
book are correct. Readers must therefore always check the product information and
clinical procedures with the most up-to-date published product information and data
sheets provided by the manufacturers and the most recent codes of conduct and
safety regulations. The authors and the publisher do not accept any liability for any
errors in the text or for the misuse or misapplication of material in this work.**

Project manager: Gavin Smith, GPS Publishing Solutions, Herts, UK
Illustrations by Graeme Chambers, BA(Hons) and Phoenix Photosetting, Chatham, Kent, UK
Typeset by Phoenix Photosetting, Chatham, Kent, UK
Printed and bound by Marston Book Services Ltd, Abingdon, Oxon, UK

Contents

Foreword

John Wilding and Sumer Aditya's book has come at a time when there is an overwhelming focus on obesity, with hundreds of new and often conflicting analyses relating to its significance, ranging from whether there are simple methods for assessing body fatness to how much significance should be given to the many varied consequences of weight gain. An even bigger muddle arises when considering how to manage overweight and obese patients, with an extra dimension now being added by the recent withdrawal of two potentially very valuable drugs which aided long term weight management. For any healthcare professional, whether based in primary or secondary care, the profusion of specific claims and analyses relating to obesity is daunting. This leads to a sense of frustration and the subsequent avoidance of obesity as an issue that ought to be dealt with as part of general clinical care. For all professionals, including doctors, nutritionists, dietitians and exercise specialists, as well as the public anxious to understand the issues, there is a further problem in that so much of the media's attention is taken up with quirky ideas and isolated findings. On this basis it is no wonder that confusion reigns as the epidemic grows worse.

This book has clearly benefited from the authors' many years of practical experience in managing obesity, and in teaching both medical students and postgraduates from a wide range of disciplines who have been attending the annual Liverpool postgraduate course in obesity management. The use of multiple diagrams to illustrate the different concepts in each chapter clearly comes from hands-on experience of how best to communicate what are sometimes quite complicated topics.

The importance of new approaches to obesity management has clearly gone up the priority list for all those involved in health care. This in part stems from the Ministers of Health meeting in Istanbul in November 2006, when 53 nations were called on by the European Region of the World Health Organisation to do something practical about the economically unsustainable explosion of obesity. For the first time, the Ministers not only agreed that preventive initiatives were needed, but formally undertook to tackle the existing challenge of hundreds of millions of adults and children who needed assessment and help in coping with their overweight and obesity-related problems. Since then new analyses have clearly shown that doctors working with additional help can provide by far the most cost-effective means of coping with the national health burden. This book provides the basis for a new approach to the appropriate assessment of the overweight patient and a coherent progressive approach to improving their care and well-being on a long term basis. Only ten years ago obesity was described as the biggest unrecognised public health problem confronting the world: the authors are to be congratulated on providing a practical book that may help health care professionals tackle this major disorder.

Philip James
April, 2011

Preface

We are in the middle of twin epidemics of obesity and type 2 diabetes, which are certainly inter-related. The awareness of obesity as a major healthcare concern has grown rapidly in the last decade and obesity has been aptly labelled as 'the millennium disease'. Obesity is not only one of the major modifiable risk factors for cardiovascular disease and death, but also contributes to the development of many other serious health disorders such as type 2 diabetes, metabolic syndrome, obstructive sleep apnoea, respiratory disease, musculoskeletal disease and many common cancers. As well as these physical co-morbidities, obesity is associated with a significant burden of psychological disease and adverse social consequences, resulting in impaired quality of life, reduced productivity and additional costs to already over-burdened health care systems. The cost to society for current and future generations is likely to be immense.

Despite the increasing awareness of the seriousness and scale of the obesity epidemic, currently available educational resources and material available are limited. This atlas has been produced with the aim of providing an accessible and practical summary of the epidemiology, aetiology, complications and management of obesity, placed in the context of recent scientific and clinical developments, which should be essential background information for everyone interested in obesity.

The initial section describes the common methods of defining and stratifying obesity and briefly discusses the epidemiology of this condition which was initially considered a disease of affluent society, but is now recognised to be a universal problem, increasingly affecting the developing world and lower socio-economic classes. The pathophysiology and aetiology of obesity is complex and multi-factorial; we have discussed energy balance, appetite regulation, genetic influence and the effect of modern lifestyle and environmental factors. The growing interests in foetal and infant origins of obesity in addition to secondary causes of obesity are also highlighted.

We have discussed the associations and complications of obesity which are immense and significant. Over the last few decades, body weight has been identified as a major risk factor affecting almost all body organs and physiological systems. We have summarised some of the latest research in this field, with appropriates figures and tables, and also provided references for further reading. Obesity management is often difficult and needs to be multi-dimensional. We have discussed the role of lifestyle modification with details of common types of dietary, exercise and behavioural interventions. There has been a huge interest in pharmacological treatment of obesity but the current options are limited. We have highlighted the past experiences and the difficulties in finding an effective yet safe therapeutic agent. The risk of adverse effects has limited these options and has lead to withdrawal of previously approved agents that initially showed great promise. Bariatric surgery, although an expensive option with limited availability, has become very popular in the last decade and we have discussed the types of procedures used in the world today. Long-term data about the risks and benefits of each surgery type are provided, along with details of prognosis and mortality.

Tackling this epidemic requires strategic planning and implementation at various levels. We have discussed, in the final section, the barriers and solutions to effective care of obesity and prevention of this modern, lifestyle-related, public health concern. Obviously there is a great deal of interest in obesity amongst researchers, clinicians, the pharmaceutical industry and surgeons to understand the pathophysiology and consequences of obesity and to develop safe and effective treatment of this common disorder. We have summarised some of the advances in this area, with particular interest in future of obesity pharmacotherapy, genetic research, functional neuro-imaging and have discussed newer bariatric surgical procedures and techniques which promise to be more effective and less invasive.

We hope this atlas will provide up-to-date and easily accessible information to people from various disciplines who are interested in obesity. The atlas is full of easy to understand figures and tables with concise written material which will be of use to clinicians, allied health professionals and students alike. All sections in the atlas are referenced, to easily direct readers towards further reading material and recent scientific developments. More work is urgently needed to tackle this huge epidemic and we hope this atlas is one small step in that direction.

Bhandari Sumer Aditya
John PH Wilding
April 2011

Acknowledgements

Dr Paul Albert
Consultant in Respiratory Medicine
University Hospital Aintree
Liverpool, UK

Dr Daniel Cuthbertson
Senior Lecturer and Honorary Consultant Physician
University Hospital Aintree
Liverpool, UK

Dr Christina Daousi
Senior Lecturer and Honorary Consultant Physician
University Hospital Aintree
Liverpool, UK

Abbreviations

5-HT	5-hydroxytryptamine/serotonin
ADA	American Diabetes Association
AgRP	Agouti-related peptide
AHA	American Heart Association
AMI	acute myocardial infarction
α-MSH	alpha-melanocyte-stimulating hormone
Apo	apolipoprotein
ARCN	arcuate nucleus
BMI	body mass index
BMR	basal metabolic rate
BOLD	blood oxygen level-dependent
BP	blood pressure
BPD	biliopancreatic diversion
CART	cocaine and amphetamine-regulated transcript
CBF	cerebral blood flow
CBT	cognitive behaviour therapy
CCK	cholecystokinin
CDC	Centers for Disease Control and Prevention
CHD	coronary heart disease
CI	confidence interval
CPAP	continuous positive-airway pressure
CRESCENDO	Comprehensive Rimonabant Evaluation Study of Cardiovascular Endpoints and Outcomes
CRF	chronic renal failure
CRH	corticotrophin-releasing hormone
CRP	C-reactive protein
CT	computed tomography
CV	cardiovascular
CVD	cardiovascular disease
DB	double-blind
DBP	diastolic blood pressure
DEXA/DXA	dual energy X-ray absorptiometry
DJB	duodenal-jejunal bypass
DMN	dorsomedial nucleus
DS	duodenal switch
DSM-IV	Diagnostic and Statistical Manual of Mental Disorders, 4th Edition
DVT	deep vein thrombosis
ECS	endocannabinoid system
EDJT	endoluminal duodeno-jejunal tube
EMA	European Medicines Agency
FDA	US Food and Drug Administration
FEV_1	forced expiratory volume in 1 second
FFA	free fatty acid
fMRI	functional magnetic resonance imaging
FPG	fasting plasma glucose
FTO	fat mass and obesity-associated gene
FVC	forced vital capacity
GDM	gestational diabetes mellitus
GIANT	Genetic Investigation of Anthropometric Traits study
GFR	glomerular filtration rate
GI	gastrointestinal/glycaemic index
GIR	glucose infusion rate
GLP-1	glucagon-like peptide-1
GLUT4	glucose transporter protein-4
HbA_{1c}	glycosylated haemoglobin
HDL	high-density lipoprotein
HDL-C	high-density lipoprotein cholesterol
HES	Hospital Episode Statistics
HF	heart failure
$HOMA_{IR}$	homeostasis model of assessment–insulin resistance
HR	heart rate
HTN	hypertension
IARC	International Agency for Research on Cancer
IASO	International Association for the Study of Obesity
ICAM-1	intercellular adhesion molecule-1
ICD-10	International Statistical Classification of Diseases and Related Health Problems, 10th Revision
IDF	International Diabetes Federation
IGB	intragastric balloon
IGT	impaired glucose tolerance
IL-6	interleukin-6
INSIG2	insulin induced gene 2
IOTF	International Obesity Task Force
IT	ileal interposition
ITT	intent to treat

LAGB	laparoscopic adjustable gastric banding
LDL	low-density lipoprotein
LDL-C	low-density lipoprotein cholesterol
LEPR	leptin receptor
LH	luteinising hormone
LHN	lateral hypothalamic nucleus
LOCF	last observation carried forward
LSCS	lower segment Caesarean section
LVH	left ventricular hypertrophy
MAO	monoamine oxidase
MC4R	melanocortin-4 receptor
MCH-1	melanin-concentrating hormone-1
MCP-1	monocyte chemoattractant protein-1
MET	metabolic equivalent
MI	myocardial infarction
MRFIT	Multiple Risk Factor Intervention Trial
MRI	magnetic resonance imaging
MRS	magnetic resonance spectroscopy
Na	sodium
NASH	non-alcoholic steatohepatitis
NCEP-ATP III	Third Report of the National Cholesterol Education Program
ND	not determined
NEAT	non-exercise activity thermogenesis
NEFA	non-esterified fatty acids
NFS	National Food Survey (UK)
NHANES	National Health and Nutrition Examination Survey
NHLBI	National Heart, Lung and Blood Institute
NOTES	natural orifice transluminal endoscopic surgery
NP	natriuretic peptide
NPY	neuropeptide-Y
OA	osteoarthritis
ODST	overnight dexamethasone suppression test
OFC	orbitofrontal cortex
OGTT	oral glucose tolerance test
OHS	obesity hypoventilation syndrome
OSA	obstructive sleep apnoea
OSAS	obstructive sleep apnoea syndrome
OTC	over-the-counter
PAF	population attributable fraction
PAI-1	plasminogen activator inhibitor-1
PAR	population attributable risk
PCOS	polycystic ovarian syndrome
PET	positron emission tomography
PFC	prefrontal cortex
PHLA	post-heparin lipolytic activity

POMC	proopiomelanocortin
PP	postprandial
PVN	paraventricular nucleus
PVR	peripheral vascular resistance
PYY	peptide YY
QOL	quality of life
QTL	quantitative trait locus
RAAS	renin–angiotensin–aldosterone system
RAPSODI	Rimonabant in Prediabetic Subjects to Delay Onset of Type 2 Diabetes study
RBP-4	retinol binding protein-4
rCBF	regional cerebral blood flow
RIO-Diabetes	Rimonabant in Obesity – Diabetes study
RIO-Europe	Rimonabant in Obesity – Europe study
RIO-Lipids	Rimonabant in Obesity – Lipids study
RIO-North America	Rimonabant in Obesity – North America study
ROS	reactive oxygen species
RR	relative risk
RYGB	Roux-en-Y gastric bypass
SB	single-blind
SBP	systolic blood pressure
SCOUT	Sibutramine Cardiovascular Outcomes trial
SEM	standard error of the mean
SERENADE	Study Evaluating Rimonabant Efficacy in Drug-Naive Diabetic Patients
SG	sleeve gastrectomy
SHBG	sex hormone-binding globulin
SHIELD	Study to Help Improve Early evaluation and management of risk factors Leading to Diabetes
SN	supra-optic nucleus
SNP	single nucleotide polymorphism
SNS	sympathetic nervous system
STORM	Sibutramine Trial of Obesity Reduction and Maintenance
TBW	total body water
TG	triglyceride
TNF-α	tumour necrosis factor-alpha
UWW	underwater weighing
VLCD	very low calorie diet
VLDL	very low-density lipoprotein cholesterol
VMN	ventromedial nucleus
WC	waist circumference
WHO	Word Health Organization
WHR	waist-to-hip ratio
XENDOS	XENical in the Prevention of Diabetes in Obese Subjects

Chapter 1

Obesity

Definition, classification, and measurements

Obesity can be defined in simple terms as the excessive amount of body fat associated with an increased risk of medical illnesses and premature death. It is the result of a complex process of undesirable positive energy balance and weight gain. Although the total body fat mass is important, it is now recognized that the localization of excess fat, particularly intra-abdominal and visceral fat, has a stronger correlation with risk of diabetes and cardiovascular disease (CVD).[1] The risk of coexisting diseases associated with obesity is also affected by a range of factors, including nature of the diet, ethnic group, and activity level.

Body mass index (BMI) is a simple index of 'weight-for-height'. The calculation of BMI is shown in **1.1**. Clinically, 'obesity' is defined as a BMI of ≥30 kg/m². Overweight is defined as a BMI of between 25 and 30 kg/m² (*Table 1.1*).

Body Mass Index (BMI) = Weight in kg / Height in metres²
Body Mass Index (BMI) = Weight in pounds × 703 / Height in inches²

1.1 Calculation of BMI.

Markers of increased risk are as follows:

1. Waist circumference >102 cm (40 inches) in men and >88 cm (35 inches) in women.
2. Weight gain of ≥5 kg since age 18–20 years.
3. Poor aerobic fitness.
4. Certain ethnic groups (e.g. South Asian, Pacific islanders, Pima Indians).

Although BMI measurements can sometimes be misleading (e.g. muscular individuals, old age, ethnic variations), there appears to be a good correlation between BMI and the percentage of body fat.[4] There is also a strong correlation between BMI and mortality (**1.2**).[5]

Table 1.1 Classification of obesity in adults according to BMI and risk of obesity-related diseases[2,3]

	Obesity class	BMI (kg/m²)	Associated risk
Underweight		<18.5	Low (but risk of other health problems increased)
Normal		18.5–24.9	Normal
Overweight	Pre-obese	25.0–29.9	Increased
Obesity	I	30.0–34.9	Moderate
	II	35.0–39.9	Severe
Extreme obesity	III	≥40.0	Very severe

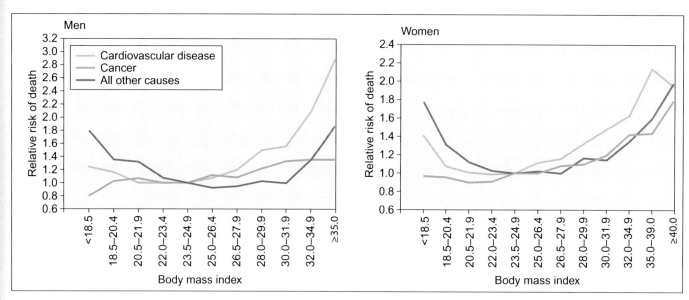

1.2 Association between BMI and cardiovascular mortality (with permission[5]).

Table 1.2 Health risk associated with overweight and obesity in adults based on BMI and waist circumference[6]

BMI classification	Waist circumference		
	Low	**High**	**Very high**
Overweight	No increased risk	Increased risk	High risk
Obesity Class I	Increased risk	High risk	Very high risk

For men, waist circumference <94 cm is low, 94–102 cm is high and >102 cm is very high.
For women, waist circumference <80 cm is low, 80–88 cm is high and >88 cm is very high.

In people with a BMI <35 kg/m[2], further classification based on a combination of BMI and waist circumference is useful in identifying those at increased risk of comorbidities (*Table 1.2*).[6]

The BMI cut-off points used to classify obesity are arbitrary along a continuum of increasing risk with increasing BMI. However, these associations are based on epidemiological data from largely Caucasian populations. In some ethnic groups such as the Asia Pacific population, the risk of comorbidities and mortality is greater at much lower BMI levels (**1.3**).[7,8] There is also an increased tendency to accumulate intra-abdominal fat without developing generalized obesity.[9] Therefore, an alternate classification of weight by BMI for adult Asians has been proposed in the World Health Organization/International Association for the Study of Obesity/International Obesity Task Force (WHO/IASO/

IOTF) Asia Pacific report (*Table 1.3*).[10] It is, however, difficult to apply the same cut-off points for all Asian subpopulations and several recommendations have been made to identify the high-risk groups by the WHO expert consultation.[11]

In children, adiposity measures are dependent on their stage of maturation. Therefore, the BMI in childhood changes substantially with age. Several countries use their own age- and gender-specific BMI charts; furthermore, the BMI cut-off used to define overweight and obesity in children also varies by country. A generally accepted cut-off to define overweight in children has been a BMI above the 95th percentile on the chart appropriate for the child's gender (*Table 1.4*). In order to facilitate global comparisons of trends in childhood and adolescent obesity rates, the IOTF developed standardized BMI centile curves that define cut-off points related to age to define childhood overweight/obesity (**1.4**).[12]

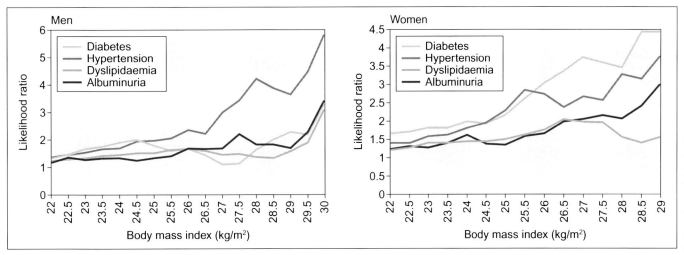

1.3 Risk of diabetes, hypertension, dyslipidaemia or albuminuria according to selected BMI cut-offs in Hong Kong Chinese men (A) and women (B) (with permission[8]).

Table 1.3 Proposed classification of weight by BMI in adult Asians[10]

Classification	BMI (kg/m²)	Risk of comorbidities
Underweight	<18.5	Low (but increased risk of other health problems)
Normal range	18.5–22.9	Average
Overweight	≥23	
At risk	23–24.9	Increased
Obese I	25–29.9	Moderate
Obese II	≥30	Severe

Additional risk: waist circumference ≥90 cm in men and ≥80 cm in women.

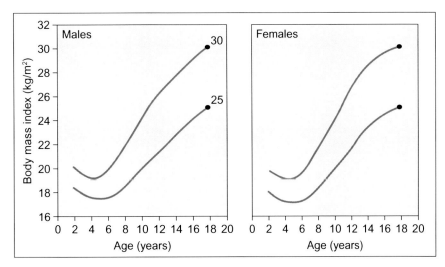

1.4 International cut-off points for BMI by sex for overweight and obesity, passing through body mass index 25 and 30 kg/m² at age 18 (data from Brazil, Great Britain, Hong Kong, The Netherlands, Singapore and the United States) (with permission[12]).

Table 1.4 Classification of obesity in children (between 2 and 20 years of age)

	BMI (kg/m²)
Underweight	<5th percentile for age and sex
Normal weight	Between 5th and 85th percentile for age and sex
Overweight	Between 85th and 95th percentile for age and sex
Obese	≥95th percentile for age and sex

Body composition: body fat content and fat distribution

While BMI is useful in classification of obesity, it has several limitations; it does not accurately estimate the body fat content in all populations or give information about fat distribution. Several techniques such as underwater weighing (UWW), air displacement plethysmography using the BOD POD®, bioelectrical impedance, and dual energy X-ray absorptiometry (DEXA) analysis are often used in research settings to measure total body fat content, whereas imaging using computed tomography (CT) and magnetic resonance imaging (MRI) are used to study fat distribution. However, most of these are expensive and impractical for routine clinical use. Simple anthropometric measurements can be used in clinical practice for this purpose.

Anthropometric measurements
Waist circumference
Waist circumference is a simple means of estimating overall adiposity and also correlates better with intra-abdominal fat content than BMI alone. It is measured (preferably after an overnight fast) directly over the skin at the end of normal expiration, horizontally, midway between the lower costal margin and the iliac crest with the arms relaxed at the sides. High waist circumference is associated with increased diabetes and cardiovascular (CV) risk independent of BMI, age, and ethnicity (**1.5**, *Table 1.5*).

Waist-to-hip ratio
This has been used as a further measure of fat distribution. Hip circumference is measured horizontally over the widest parts of the gluteal region. Waist-to-hip ratio (WHR) is then calculated. A WHR >0.95 in men and >0.80 in women is said to be indicative of central obesity. Although it correlates well with disease risk, the change in WHR is less remarkable than waist circumference alone with weight change and is, therefore, less useful in clinical practice (**1.6–1.9**).

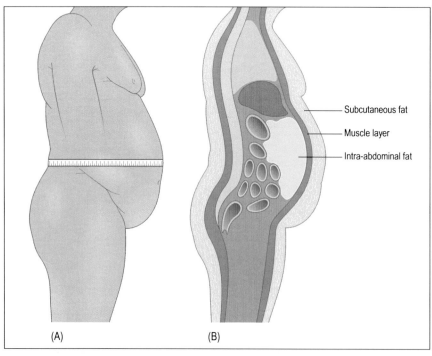

1.5 (A) Measurement of waist circumference and (B) distribution of intra-abdominal fat.

Table 1.5 Adjusted odds ratios for metabolic diseases comparing high versus normal waist circumference within different body mass index categories[13]

	Normal weight		Overweight		Class 1 obese	
	Men	**Women**	**Men**	**Women**	**Men**	**Women**
Hypertension	2.26	1.87	1.47	2.04	1.09	15.85
Type 2 diabetes	2.16	1.52	1.99	4.07	0.97	14.82
Hypercholesterolaemia	1.31	1.71	1.48	1.43	0.91	2.27
High LDL cholesterol level	1.71	1.67	1.31	1.50	0.71	29.17
Low LDL cholesterol level	0.54	1.93	1.55	1.46	1.80	2.27
Hypertriglyceridaemia	0.93	3.11	1.90	1.90	1.55	2.04
Metabolic syndrome	0.67	1.76	2.13	2.20	2.90	28.60

LDL, low-density lipoprotein.

Abdominal sagittal diameter

Abdominal sagittal diameter is measured as the distance between the examination table and the highest point of the abdomen, with the subject in a supine position (**1.10**). Although the sagittal diameter shows the strongest relationship to intra-abdominal fat mass of all the anthropometric measurements, there are currently insufficient data to support its general use.

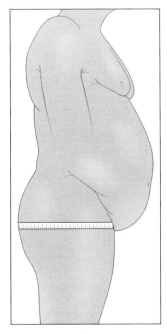

1.6 Measurement of hip circumference.

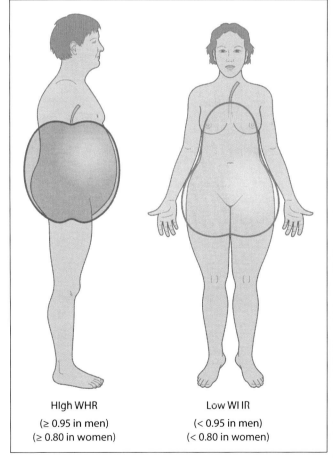

High WHR
(≥ 0.95 in men)
(≥ 0.80 in women)

Low WHR
(< 0.95 in men)
(< 0.80 in women)

1.7 Schematic demonstration of 'apple shaped' (upper body, android or abdominal obesity) and 'pear shaped' (lower body, gynoid or peripheral obesity) phenotypes based on WHR measurements.

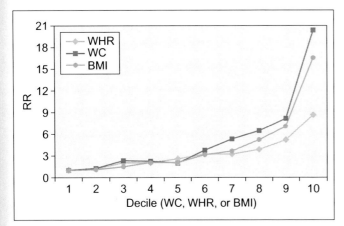

1.8 Graph showing the association between anthropometric measurements and age-adjusted relative risk (RR) of type 2 diabetes by baseline waist circumference (WC), waist-to-hip ratio (WHR), and BMI deciles. A prospective cohort study (Health Professionals Follow-Up Study) of 27 270 men with a 13-year follow-up (with permission[14]).

Measurement of body composition
Skinfold thickness
Subcutaneous fat is measured at several sites using standard callipers and can predict total fat mass with reasonable accuracy. The commonly used sites are triceps, biceps, anterior thigh, sub-scapular, and supra-iliac areas. These measurements are age- and gender-specific and can be used to predict body density and total body fat. However, they are prone to inter- and intra-observer variations and, therefore, not recommended for routine clinical use. They can be used in research studies along with other measures of adiposity, and to monitor progressive changes *within* individuals.

Bioelectrical impedance
This method is based on the principle that fat is a poor conductor of applied current whereas fat-free tissue, due to its water and electrolyte content, is a good electrical conductor. A small current is passed through the body to measure the body

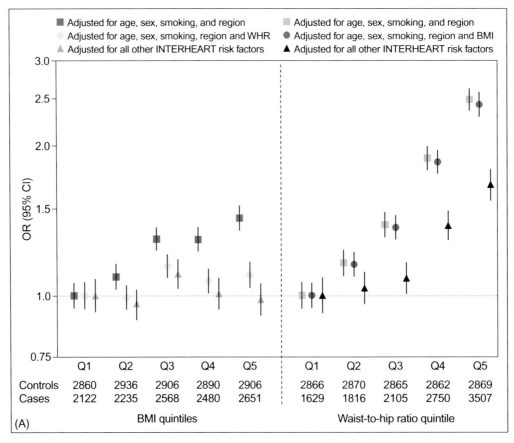

1.9 Association between anthropometric measurements and risk of acute myocardial infarction. Obesity and the risk of myocardial infarction in 27 000 participants from 52 countries: a case–control study. (A) Association of BMI and waist-to-hip ratio with myocardial infarction risk.

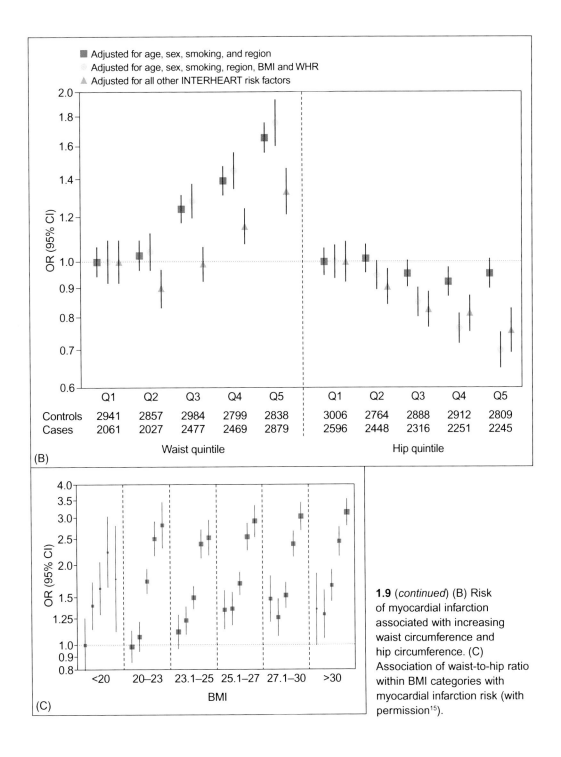

Adjusted for age, sex, smoking, and region
Adjusted for age, sex, smoking, region, BMI and WHR
Adjusted for all other INTERHEART risk factors

(B)

	Q1	Q2	Q3	Q4	Q5	Q1	Q2	Q3	Q4	Q5
Controls	2941	2857	2984	2799	2838	3006	2764	2888	2912	2809
Cases	2061	2027	2477	2469	2879	2596	2448	2316	2251	2245

Waist quintile   Hip quintile

(C)

BMI

1.9 (*continued*) (B) Risk of myocardial infarction associated with increasing waist circumference and hip circumference. (C) Association of waist-to-hip ratio within BMI categories with myocardial infarction risk (with permission[15]).

impedance. The bioelectrical impedance analysis of body water is used to estimate body fat and fat-free (lean) mass (**1.11**A, B). In spite of several limitations, these techniques offer a better estimation of fat content, have less observer error than anthropometric measurements, and can be useful for monitoring changes *within* individuals in clinical practice.

Air displacement plethysmography (BOD POD®)
The BOD POD® uses patented 'air displacement technology' for determining percentage fat and fat-free mass in adults and children. The simple, 5-minute test consists of measuring the subject's mass (weight) using a very accurate electronic scale, and volume, which is determined by sitting inside the

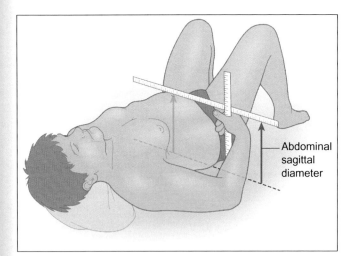

Abdominal
sagittal
diameter

1.10 Measurement of abdominal sagittal diameter. Abdominal sagittal diameter is commonly assessed using a sagittometer (i.e. a sliding beam calliper with a ruler). Sagittal diameter should be measured at the end of a normal expiration while the individual is relaxed and in a supine position. To measure sagittal diameter, place one of the callipers under the individual's back and close the other calliper until it touches the highest part of the abdomen. The callipers should be perpendicular to the ground. The callipers should be snug without indenting the individual's skin.

BOD POD® chamber. From these two measurements, the subject's body composition is calculated (**1.11**C, D).

The BOD POD® consists of the front (or test) chamber, where the subject sits, and a reference chamber. A diaphragm in the common wall oscillates during testing causing small volume changes. The pressure response to these changes in volume is measured. This is done by measuring the interior volume of the empty BOD POD® chamber, then measuring it again when the subject is seated inside. By subtraction, the subject's body volume is obtained.

Once the subject's mass and volume are determined, body density is calculated and the relative proportions of fat and fat-free mass are determined. This procedure is more user-friendly than UWW, can accommodate heavier patients than DEXA, CT, or MRI machines, and there is no radiation exposure. However, the equipment is too expensive for routine clinical use. A smaller version is available for the measurement of body composition in babies and very young children (PEAPOD®).

Dual energy X-ray absorptiometry
DEXA uses an X-ray beam with two energy peaks (high and low) in combination with a whole body scanner. This method is able to differentiate fat mass, fat-free mass, and bone mineral mass for the total body or for specific anatomic regions through the differential absorption of the high- and low-energy X-rays by these various tissues (**1.12**). There is a small radiation exposure, but measurements are very precise and reliable. DEXA scanners are widely available in healthcare settings as they are frequently used to measure bone mineral density to asses the risk of osteoporosis (an additional software package is required to assess body composition). It is also very useful in the assessment of adiposity in children but is not recommended for routine clinical use.

Imaging techniques: computed tomography and magnetic resonance imaging
These can provide a direct measure of fat distribution, typically in the abdominal region (**1.13**). It is possible to discriminate between subcutaneous and intra-abdominal deposits (omental, mesenteric, and retroperitoneal), which may be associated with independent metabolic effects. There is good correlation between the fat areas measured in a single CT/MRI slice at the level of L4–L5 with total visceral fat volume.[16] Magnetic resonance spectroscopy (MRS) techniques are now being used to determine visceral fat distribution accurately. Their use is limited by availability, cost, radiation exposure (CT), and the capacity of machines to accommodate very obese subjects.

Multi-compartment models
Classical methods to measure body composition are based on the two-compartment model, in which the body is assumed to be composed of fat and fat-free tissue. UWW, total body water (TBW), bioelectrical impedance, or skinfold thickness are all based on the assumption that the composition of fat-free mass is constant. However, this is not reliable in certain groups such as children, the elderly, and physically fit individuals. Multi-compartment models have been used to overcome these limitations.

The multi-compartment model used to measure body composition requires a combination of measurement methods.

1. Determination of total body water by using deuterium or ^{18}O-labelled water dilution.
2. Body mass.
3. Body volume by air displacement (BOD POD®) or UWW.
4. Bone mineral content by DEXA.

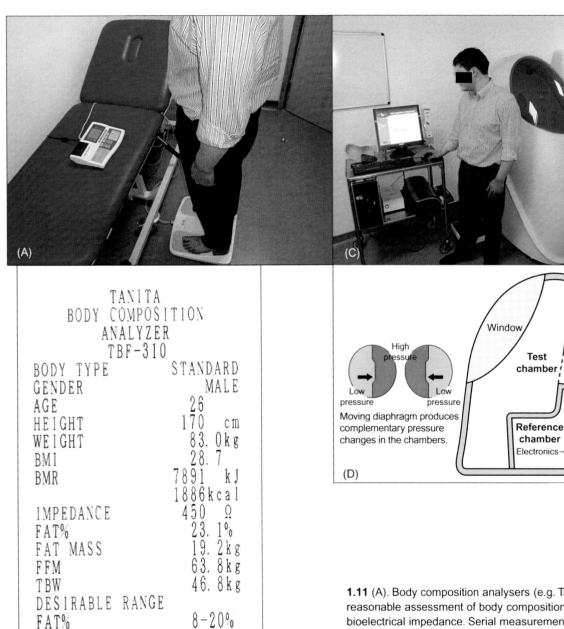

TANITA
BODY COMPOSITION
ANALYZER
TBF-310

BODY TYPE	STANDARD
GENDER	MALE
AGE	26
HEIGHT	170 cm
WEIGHT	83.0 kg
BMI	28.7
BMR	7891 kJ
	1886 kcal
IMPEDANCE	450 Ω
FAT%	23.1%
FAT MASS	19.2 kg
FFM	63.8 kg
TBW	46.8 kg
DESIRABLE RANGE	
FAT%	8-20%
FAT MASS	5.6-16.0 kg

(B)

(A)

(C)

Window   Diaphragm

High pressure

Test chamber   Computer

Low pressure   Low pressure

Moving diaphragm produces complementary pressure changes in the chambers.

Reference chamber

Electronics→   Scale

(D)

1.11 (A). Body composition analysers (e.g. Tanita) provide a reasonable assessment of body composition by measuring bioelectrical impedance. Serial measurements are useful in a clinical setting to monitor progress. (B) Example printout from the Tanita body composition analyser. (C, D) Measurement of body composition using BOD POD®.

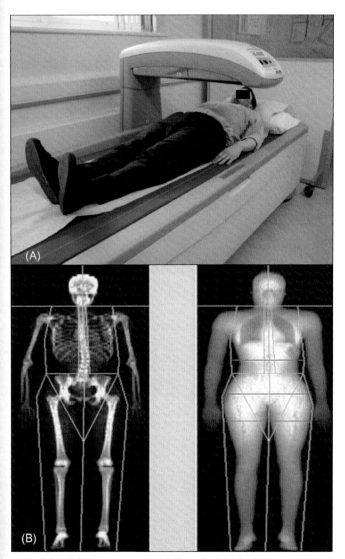

1.12 Using DEXA measurements to calculate body composition.

1.13 (A) MRI image of cross-section of abdomen showing distribution of abdominal fat. In the coloured version of the same image (B), green = subcutaneous fat and red = intra-abdominal fat.

Epidemiology

The World Health Organization has agreed a general classification of weight, based on BMI (see earlier section in this chapter). Lower cut-off points are recommended in some populations because of increased disease risk at a lower BMI level, but a generalized classification allows estimation and comparison of global and regional obesity rates. However, the global perspective on obesity is very complex and there are several factors that could explain the large differences between populations in the distribution of BMI:

1. Demographic factors: age distribution; gender; and ethnicity.
2. Socio-cultural factors: educational level; economic status; and marital status.
3. Biological factors: parity and family history
4. Behavioural factors: dietary habits; smoking; alcohol consumption; and physical activity and lifestyle.

Recent analysis reveals marked disparities in the obesity prevalence rates among different countries within regions, as well as substantial differences in prevalence of obesity within the developing world. Traditionally, obesity was seen as a sign of affluence but now, in both developed and developing countries, obesity is particularly marked in the lower socio-economic classes. Throughout the world, women in general have a higher prevalence of obesity, but more men are in the overweight category.

The prevalence of obesity is increasing at an alarming rate in both developed and developing countries. Of particular concern is the increase in obesity and overweight rates in children. The increase in prevalence of obesity across the world seems to be closely related to the increases in prevalence of cardiovascular disease, type 2 diabetes, and mortality. Obesity could be regarded as 'The Millennium Disease' and the epidemic may continue to rise, with serious health consequences if appropriate action is not taken to reverse current trends (**1.14–1.21**).

Recent estimates suggest that, globally, more than 1 billion adults are overweight, and at least 300 million of them are obese. Childhood obesity is already epidemic in some areas and on the rise in others. World-wide, 22 million children <5 years of age are estimated to be overweight. Obesity accounts for 2.6% of total healthcare costs in developed countries; some estimates put the figure as high as 7%. The true costs are undoubtedly much greater, as not all obesity-related conditions are included in the calculations (**1.22**).

In summary, obesity can be defined by estimates of body 'fatness', supplemented by measures of fat distribution. Obesity is now highly prevalent in most populations and predisposes to many common diseases with significant associated healthcare costs.

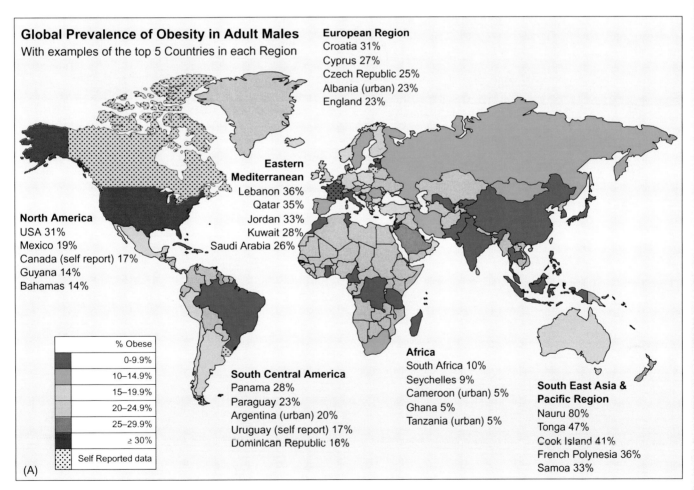

1.14 World maps showing prevalence of obesity in (A) men (with permission[17]).

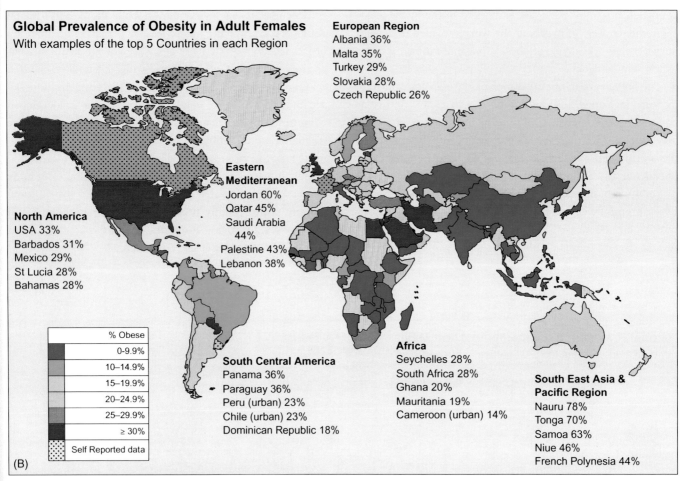

Global Prevalence of Obesity in Adult Females
With examples of the top 5 Countries in each Region

European Region
Albania 36%
Malta 35%
Turkey 29%
Slovakia 28%
Czech Republic 26%

Eastern Mediterranean
Jordan 60%
Qatar 45%
Saudi Arabia 44%
Palestine 43%
Lebanon 38%

North America
USA 33%
Barbados 31%
Mexico 29%
St Lucia 28%
Bahamas 28%

Africa
Seychelles 28%
South Africa 28%
Ghana 20%
Mauritania 19%
Cameroon (urban) 14%

South Central America
Panama 36%
Paraguay 36%
Peru (urban) 23%
Chile (urban) 23%
Dominican Republic 18%

South East Asia & Pacific Region
Nauru 78%
Tonga 70%
Samoa 63%
Niue 46%
French Polynesia 44%

% Obese
0-9.9%
10–14.9%
15–19.9%
20–24.9%
25–29.9%
≥ 30%
Self Reported data

(B)

1.14 (*continued*) and (B) women (with permission[17]).

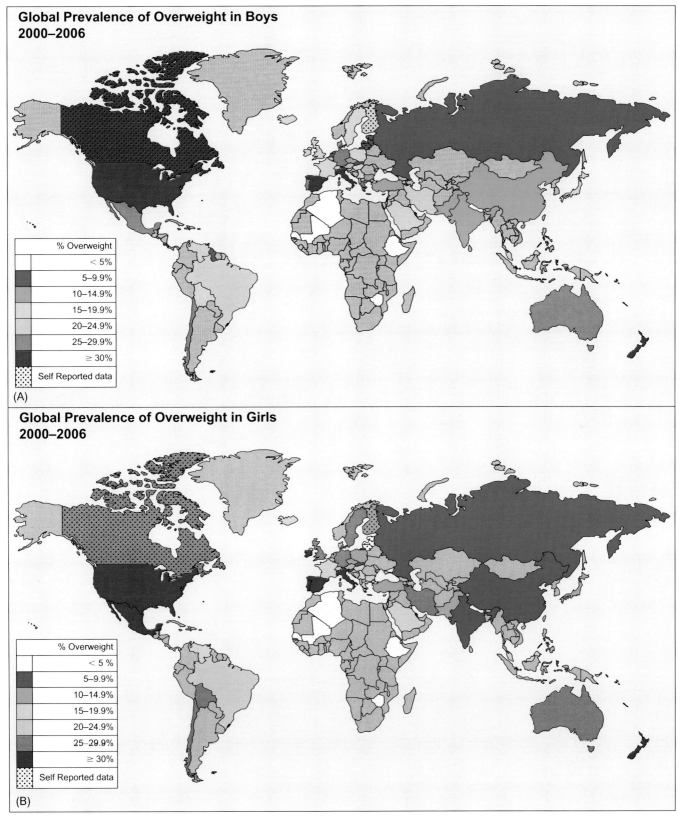

Global Prevalence of Overweight in Boys 2000–2006

% Overweight	
	< 5%
	5–9.9%
	10–14.9%
	15–19.9%
	20–24.9%
	25–29.9%
	≥ 30%
	Self Reported data

(A)

Global Prevalence of Overweight in Girls 2000–2006

% Overweight	
	< 5 %
	5–9.9%
	10–14.9%
	15–19.9%
	20–24.9%
	25–29.9%
	≥ 30%
	Self Reported data

(B)

1.15 World maps showing prevalence of obesity in (A) boys and (B) girls (with permission[17]).

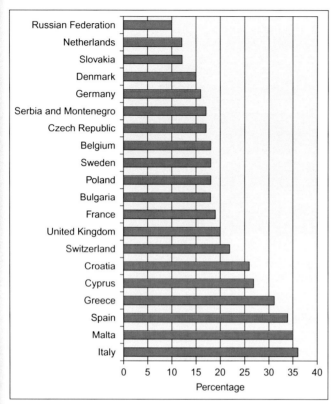

1.16 Prevalence of childhood obesity in European countries (with permission[18]).

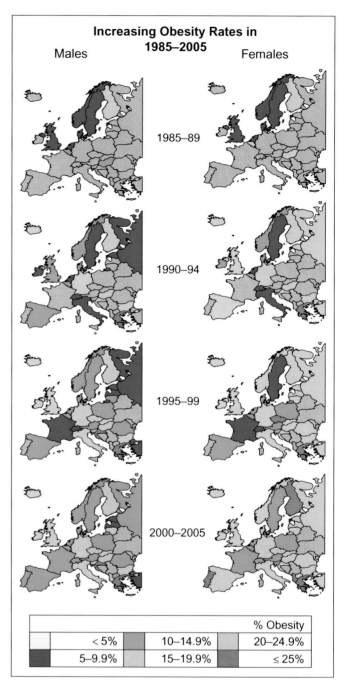

1.17 Increasing obesity rates in Europe (1985–2005) (with permission[17]).

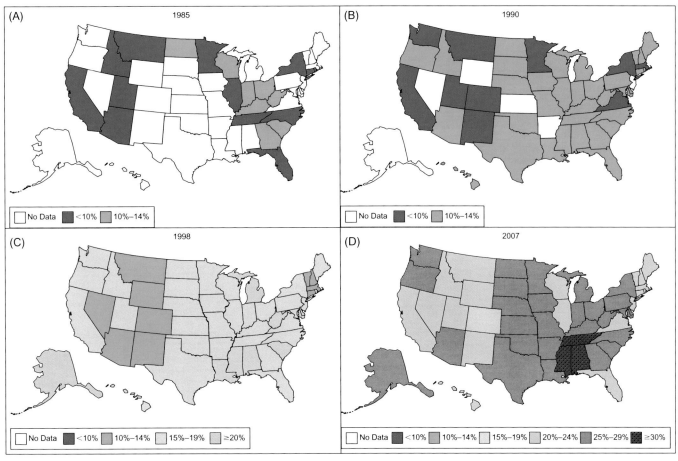

1.18 Serial US maps showing obesity rates and trends (1985–2007): BMI ≥30, or ~30 lbs. overweight for 5 ft 4 in person). Source: CDC Behavioral Risk Factor Surveillance System (with permission[19]).

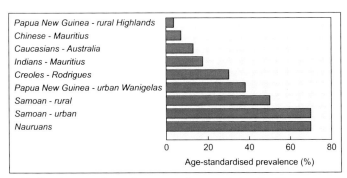

1.19 Obesity prevalence in women from an Asian Pacific population (with permission[9,10]).

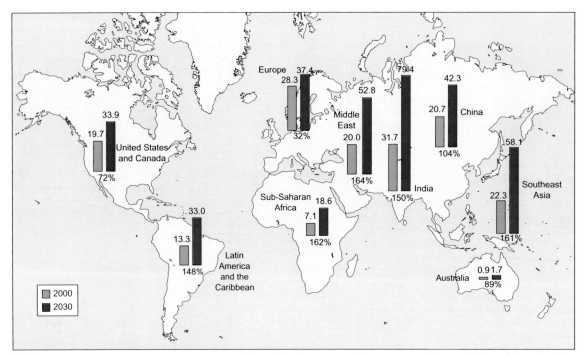

1.20 Millions of cases of diabetes in 2000 and projections for 2030, with projected percentage changes. The serious rise in prevalence of diabetes is thought to be linked to the projected increase in obesity rates in different countries[20,21] (data with permission from[21]).

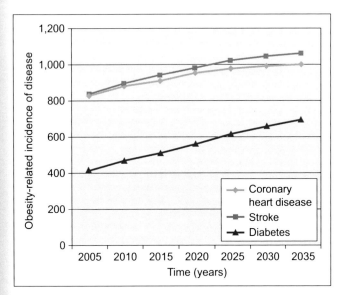

1.21 Projected prevalence of diseases attributable to obesity. The UK Government's Foresight programme, aimed at tackling obesity submitted its project report in October 2007. The impact of obesity on the incidence of coronary artery disease, stroke, and diabetes in the future was assessed using a micro-simulation that imposed the known association between BMI and health risks from the present day to 2050. The analysis indicates that the greatest increase in the incidence of disease would be for type 2 diabetes (>70% increase by 2050) with increases of 30% for stroke and 20% for ischaemic heart disease (with permission[22]).

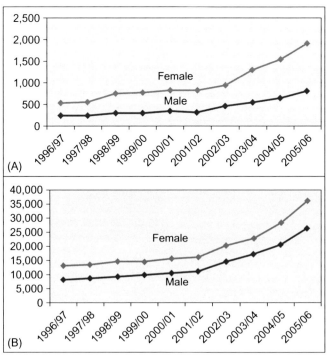

1.22 Finished consultant episodes with primary (A) and secondary (B) diagnosis of obesity in England between 1996 and 2006.[23] Data obtained from Hospital Episode Statistics, HES—The Information Centre (with permission from http://www.hesonline.org.uk).

References

1. Janssen I, Katzmarzyk PT, Ross R. Waist circumference and not body mass index explains obesity-related health risk. *Am J Clin Nutr* 2004; **79**: 379–84.
2. Clinical Guidelines on the Identification, Evaluation, and Treatment of Overweight and Obesity in Adults—The Evidence Report. National Institutes of Health. *Obes Res* 1998; **6**: 51S–209S.
3. Obesity: preventing and managing the global epidemic. Report of a WHO consultation. *World Health Organ Tech Rep Ser* 2000; **894**: i–253.
4. Deurenberg P, van der KK, Hulshof T, Evers P. Body mass index as a measure of body fatness in the elderly. *Eur J Clin Nutr* 1989; **43**: 231–6.
5. Calle EE, Thun MJ, Petrelli JM, Rodriguez C, Heath CW, Jr. Body-mass index and mortality in a prospective cohort of U.S. adults. *N Engl J Med* 1999; **341**: 1097–1105.
6. NICE clinical guideline—Obesity CG 43, Dec 2006.
7. Deurenberg P, Yap M, van Staveren WA. Body mass index and percent body fat: a meta analysis among different ethnic groups. *Int J Obes Relat Metab Disord* 1998; **22**: 1164–71.
8. Ko GT, Tang J, Chan JC, *et al.* Lower BMI cut-off value to define obesity in Hong Kong Chinese: an analysis based on body fat assessment by bioelectrical impedance. *Br J Nutr* 2001; **85**: 239–42.
9. The burden of overweight and obesity in the Asia-Pacific region. *Obes Rev* 2007; **8**: 191–6.
10. WHO/IASO/IOTF. *The Asia-Pacific Perspective: redefining obesity and its treatment.* Melbourne: Health Communications Australia; 2000.
11. Appropriate body-mass index for Asian populations and its implications for policy and intervention strategies. *Lancet* 2004; **363**: 157–63.
12. Cole TJ, Bellizzi MC, Flegal KM, Dietz WH. Establishing a standard definition for child overweight and obesity worldwide: international survey. *BMJ* 2000; **320**: 1240–3.
13. Janssen I, Katzmarzyk PT, Ross R. Body mass index, waist circumference, and health risk: evidence in support of current National Institutes of Health guidelines. *Arch Intern Med* 2002; **162**: 2074–9.
14. Wang Y, Rimm EB, Stampfer MJ, Willett WC, Hu FB. Comparison of abdominal adiposity and overall obesity in predicting risk of type 2 diabetes among men. *Am J Clin Nutr* 2005; **81**: 555–63.
15. Yusuf S, Hawken S, Ounpuu S, *et al.* Obesity and the risk of myocardial infarction in 27,000 participants from 52 countries: a case-control study. *Lancet* 2005; **366**: 1640–9.
16. Kvist H, Chowdhury B, Grangard U, Tylen U, Sjostrom L. Total and visceral adipose-tissue volumes derived from measurements with computed tomography in adult men and women: predictive equations. *Am J Clin Nutr* 1988; **48**: 1351–61.
17. International Obesity Taskforce (*http://www.iotf.org/database/TrendsEuropeanadultsthroughtimev3.htm*).
18. Lobstein T, Frelut ML. Prevalence of overweight among children in Europe. *Obes Rev* 2003; **4**: 195–200.
19. CDC Behavioural Risk Factor Surveillance System—Obesity Trends Among US Adults 1985–2007.
20. Hossain P, Kawar B, El NM. Obesity and diabetes in the developing world—a growing challenge. *N Engl J Med* 2007; **356**: 213–15.
21. Wild S, Roglic G, Green A, Sicree R, King H. Global prevalence of diabetes: estimates for the year 2000 and projections for 2030. *Diabetes Care* 2004; **27**: 1047–53.
22. McPherson K, Marsh T, Brown M. Foresight report on obesity. *Lancet* 2007; **370**: 1755.
23. Hospital Episode Statistics, HES. The Information Centre 2006.

Pathophysiology and aetiology of obesity

Energy balance

Obesity is a state of undesired positive energy balance. When energy intake exceeds energy expenditure over long periods of time (usually years), it leads to accumulation of adipose tissue with a corresponding decrease in lean body mass. Even a small positive energy balance on a daily basis can lead to weight gain; a daily excess of 100 kcal leads to an approximate increase of 5 kg of fat over 12 months or 50 kg over 10 years. The resulting weight gain is also dependent on a complex interaction of genetic, biochemical, hormonal, and environmental influences.

Obesity developing at a young age is more likely to be influenced by gene-related changes in energy balance, whereas adult onset obesity is more likely to have a strong environmental component. The degree of fat accumulation and the adverse metabolic outcomes secondary to excess fat are significantly influenced by lifestyle and ethnicity. The distribution of fat is pathophysiologically significant; for example, excess fat in the abdomen is associated with an increased risk of metabolic diseases such as cardiovascular disease and diabetes.

An individual is said to be in a state of 'energy balance', if their energy intake is equal to their energy expenditure. A 'positive energy balance' occurs when the energy expenditure does not match intake and the excess energy is stored in the body primarily as fat (2.1). The quantity and pattern of energy intake in modern society has changed progressively as a result of alterations in the availability and palatability of food. There has also been a significant change in the amount of physical activity, which is an important component of energy expenditure but the principles of energy balance remain the same. Energy balance is also tightly regulated by several neural and hormonal pathways. The tendency to gain weight gradually throughout adult life probably reflects the fact that the regulatory systems have evolved to protect against weight loss rather than prevent weight gain (2.2).

The basal metabolic rate (BMR) is the energy required to maintain normal metabolism. The thermic effect of food is the energy used in digesting and storing a meal.

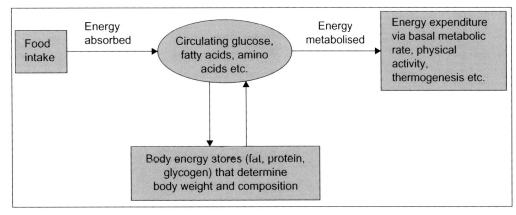

2.1 Principles of energy balance. Energy metabolism and storage is influenced by a variety of inherited (e.g. genetics), acquired (e.g. disease, drugs), and psychosocial (e.g. behavioural) factors.

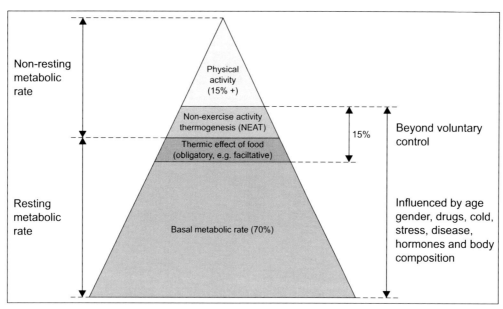

2.2 Components of energy expenditure (the energy pyramid).

This is greatest for protein in the diet, intermediate for carbohydrates and lowest for fat, which may partly explain why a high fat intake is likely to cause weight gain. Some energy is used in spontaneous and subconscious physical activity such as fidgeting, otherwise called non-exercise activity thermogenesis (NEAT). All of these components are beyond voluntary control. Energy expenditure due to voluntary physical activity is quite variable in individuals; however, obese subjects use a greater amount of energy than their lean counterparts for the same level of physical activity. Metabolic rate is also tightly coupled to energy intake. In general, metabolic rate is higher in obese than in lean individuals both at rest and during activity, dispelling the myth that obesity results from a low metabolic rate.

Appetite regulation

Much of the research into the control of energy intake focuses on the following aspects:

- Hunger and satiety control centres in the brain (**2.3**).
- Brainstem–hypothalamic neurotransmitters involved in feeding regulation.
- Hunger and satiety signals from the periphery, in particular, the gut–brain axis and peripheral adiposity signals.

It is important to understand the definition of hunger, appetite, and satiety to in turn understand the various complex appetite regulation pathways. Hunger is 'a demand for calories' (e.g. after starvation) whereas appetite refers to 'a demand for a particular food', which may or may not be proportional to the body's need for nutrition. Hunger and satiation are controlled by neural centres and related neurotransmitters; appetite and feeding patterns are strongly influenced by psychological, economic, social, and environmental factors.

Centres localized in hypothalamus that are involved in control of feeding behaviour include:

- The arcuate nucleus.
- The paraventricular nucleus.
- The ventromedial hypothalamic nucleus.
- The lateral hypothalamic nucleus.
- The perifornical area.

These centres integrate neural (vagal) and circulatory (via nutrients and hormones) signals related to the control of food intake. Neuropeptide-Y and Agouti-related peptide, expressed by neuropeptide-Y/Agouti-related peptide neurons, stimulate food intake. The proopiomelanocortin (POMC) is cleaved into α-melanocyte-stimulating hormone, which acts via melanocortin-4 receptors. Activation of the POMC/cocaine and amphetamine-regulated transcript

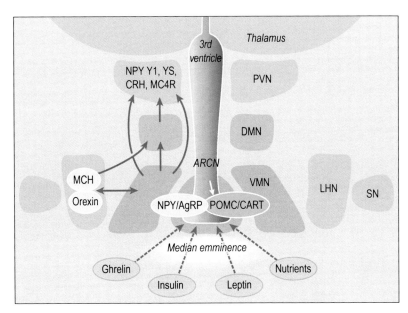

2.3 Hypothalamic circuits implicated in the control of food intake. AgRP, Agouti-related peptide; ARCN, arcuate nucleus; CART, cocaine and amphetamine-regulated transcript; CRH, corticotrophin-releasing hormone; DMN, dorsomedial nucleus; LHN, lateral hypothalamic nucleus; MC4R, melanocortin-4 receptor; MCH, melanin-concentrating hormone; NPY, neuropeptide-Y; POMC, proopiomelanocortin; PVN, paraventricular nucleus; SN, supra-optic nucleus; VMN, ventromedial nucleus.

neurons reduces food intake via the effects of α-melanocyte-stimulating hormone, cocaine and amphetamine-regulated transcript, and neurotensin. All of these neurons project to other regions in the hypothalamus, particularly in the lateral hypothalamic area, which contains neurons expressing melanin-concentrating hormone and orexins A and B, which stimulate food intake.

The gut–brain axis in appetite regulation

The passage of food through the gut initiates a number of satiety signals. The vagus nerve carries afferent signals from stretch receptors and the chemoreceptors to the hindbrain. Endocrine signals from the gut that play a part in appetite regulation are summarized in *Table 2.1*. Several peptides such as orexin, apolipoprotein A-IV, bombesin-like-peptides, enterostatin, pancreatic polypeptide, obestatin, and gastric leptin have been reported to play some part in appetite regulation and further research into their actions is awaited (**2.4**).

Skeletal muscle and adipose tissue metabolism in obesity

Skeletal muscle, which comprises 30–40% of body weight, is a major reservoir of carbohydrate and plays a significant role

Table 2.1 Gut hormones linked to appetite regulation

Gut peptide	Site of production	Main actions
Cholecystokinin	Proximal small intestine	↓ food intake
Glucagon like peptide	Ileum	↓ food intake, delay gastric emptying
Peptide YY	Ileum	↓ food intake, delay gastric emptying
Ghrelin	Stomach	↑ food intake
Amylin	Pancreatic β-cells	↓ food intake, delay gastric emptying
Oxyntomodulin	Small intestine	↓ food intake

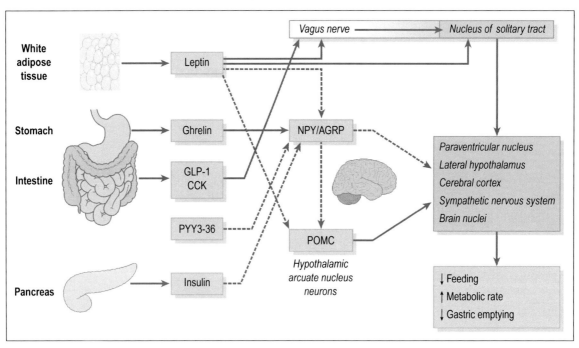

2.4 Peripheral signals involved in energy homeostasis (circulating gastrointestinal and adipocyte hormones and neuronal circuits involved in energy homeostasis: solid lines represent net stimulatory effect; dashed lines represent net inhibitory effect) (with permission[1]).

in glucose, amino acid, and lipid metabolism. Impairment of muscle oxidative metabolism can lead to accumulation of body energy stores. The most prominent defects noted in skeletal muscle metabolism in obesity are reduced utilization and storage of glucose, development of insulin resistance, and impaired fatty acid oxidation.

Metabolic consequences of increased fat deposition and fat distribution play a significant role directly and indirectly in almost all major systems and biochemical pathways. There has been a great interest in the role of non-esterified fatty acids in the development of insulin resistance. The last few decades have seen the discovery of newer adipokines, which influence metabolic pathways in the liver, skeletal muscle, gut, and brain (appetite). The role of leptin, adiponectin, resistin, visfatin, and pro-inflammatory cytokines such as interleukin-6 and tumour necrosis factor-α are being studied extensively. They not only help us understand the pathophysiology of obesity but also its consequences, such as cardiovascular disease and diabetes and they also provide potential therapeutic targets.

Leptin

This hormone is produced by adipose tissue and circulating levels reflect fat mass. Leptin receptors and downstream signalling pathways are located in the hypothalamus. Central and peripheral administration of leptin in rodents causes a profound decrease in food intake and weight loss. The ob/ob mouse, which is completely deficient in leptin, is hyperphagic, hyperinsulinaemic, and very obese. It is thought that excess leptin causes stimulation of the POMC pathway and inhibition of the neuropeptide-Y pathway resulting in decreased food intake and increased thermogenesis. Treatment of children who have rare congenital leptin deficiency with recombinant leptin has led to a significant reduction in hyperphagia and fat mass.[2] A vast majority of obese people have high leptin levels, however, and treatment with leptin does not have the same effect.

Endocannabinoid system

This is a neuromodulatory system comprising a range of molecules, synthesized from arachidonic acid precursors, which regulate synaptic neurotransmission. The stimulation of endocannabinoid receptors (CB_1 and CB_2) affects several physiological functions not only in the central nervous system but also in endocrine, reproductive, gastrointestinal, cardiovascular, and immune systems. CB_1 receptor blockade using rimonabant leads to several

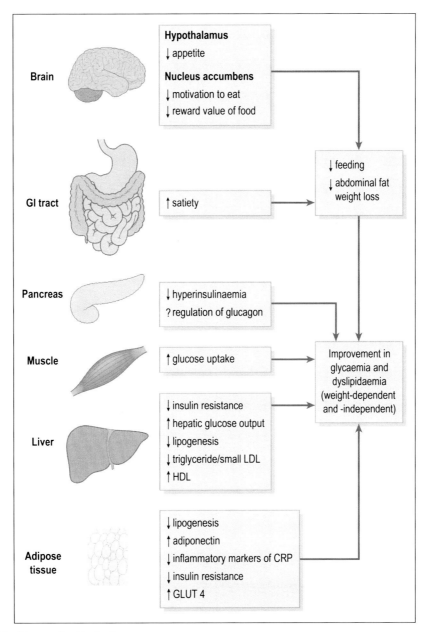

2.5 Effects of the cannabinoid receptor blockade.

beneficial metabolic changes in addition to weight loss (**2.5**). Several studies about the pathophysiological role of endocannabinoid system (ECS) and the effects of CB_1 receptor blockade are currently ongoing. Although this appears to be an exciting therapeutic target for the treatment of obesity, the recent withdrawal of rimonabant as a result of reports of neuropsychiatric side effects has tempered initial enthusiasm for manipulation of the endocannabinoid system as a potential treatment for obesity.

Genetics

Changing lifestyles and environmental factors are often quoted as the most likely explanation for the recent obesity epidemic across the globe. This does not mean that heritable factors play an insignificant role in determining the risk of weight gain. Family, adoptee, and twin studies confirm that the contribution of genetic and heritable factors to the tendency to develop obesity is about 45–75%. Progress in identifying single gene defects leading to obesity has been very slow until recently, but significant progress has been made in recent years in this field (*see* Chapter 5).

Until 2005, a series of obesity gene maps had been published (12 updates), which include all the available evidence from single gene mutation obesity cases, Mendelian disorders exhibiting obesity as a clinical feature, transgenic and knockout murine models relevant to obesity, quantitative trait loci (QTLs) from animal cross-breeding experiments, association studies with candidate genes, and linkages from genome scans. The last update was published in 2005 by Rankinen and co-workers.[3]

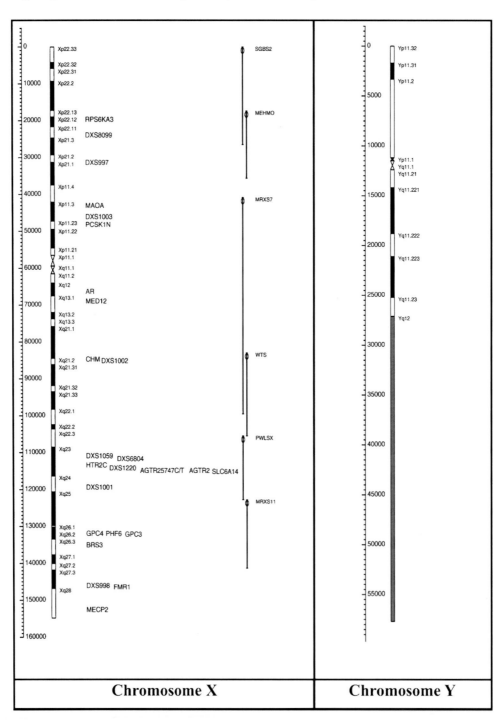

2.6 The 2005 update of human obesity gene map (with permission[3]).

This update includes 176 human obesity cases due to single gene mutations in 11 different genes, 50 loci related to Mendelian syndromes, 244 genes that, when mutated or expressed as transgenes in the mouse, result in phenotypes that affect body weight and adiposity and 408 QTLs reported from animal models (**2.6**). A total of 253 human obesity QTLs for obesity-related phenotypes from 61 genome-wide scans have been reported. The number of studies reporting associations between DNA sequence variation in specific genes and obesity phenotypes has also increased considerably, with 426 findings of positive associations with 127 candidate genes.

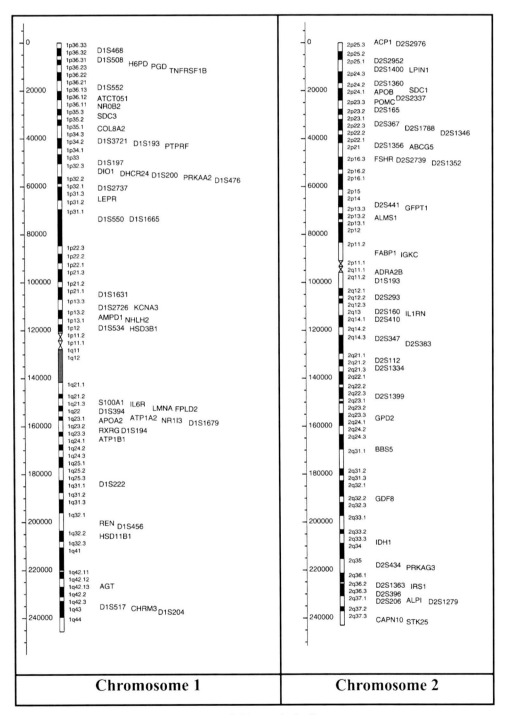

2.6 (*continued*) The 2005 update of human obesity gene map (with permission[3]).

Identification of the several gene variants and improved genetic technology in candidate gene studies has led to several interesting discoveries that are beyond the scope of this book. For example, alterations in the leptin receptor (LEPR) gene (missense or non-sense mutations) have been reported in about 3% of individuals with early onset obesity, especially those born out of consanguineous families.[2,4] Interesting

work has been done with Prader–Willi syndrome, Bardet–Beidl syndrome, leptin deficiency, POMC defects, and melanocortin-4 receptor defects, which have greatly improved our understanding of the pathophysiology of human obesity.

More recently, genetic epidemiology studies using genome-wide association techniques have led to the discovery of variants in *FTO* (fat mass and obesity-associated gene).

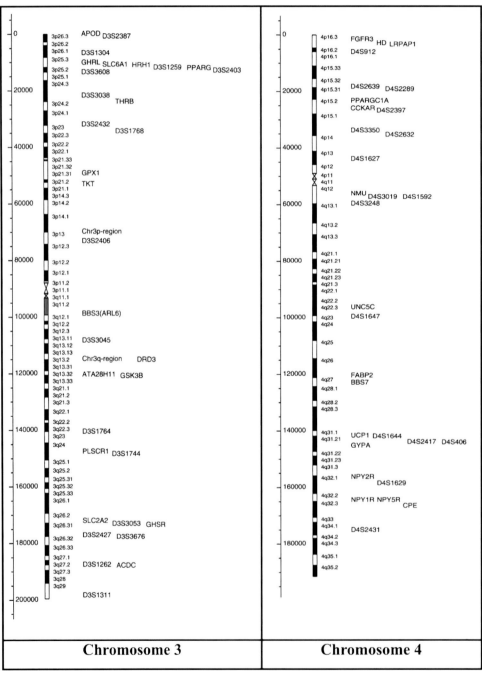

2.6 (*continued*) The 2005 update of human obesity gene map (with permission[3]).

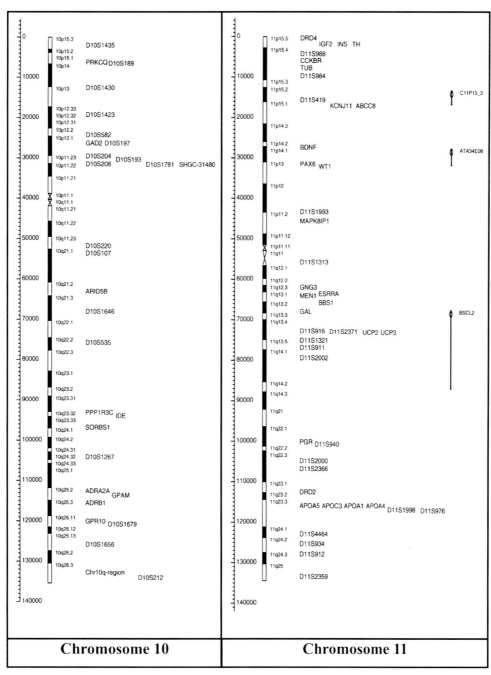

Chromosome 10

Chromosome 11

2.6 (*continued*) The 2005 update of human obesity gene map (with permission[3]).

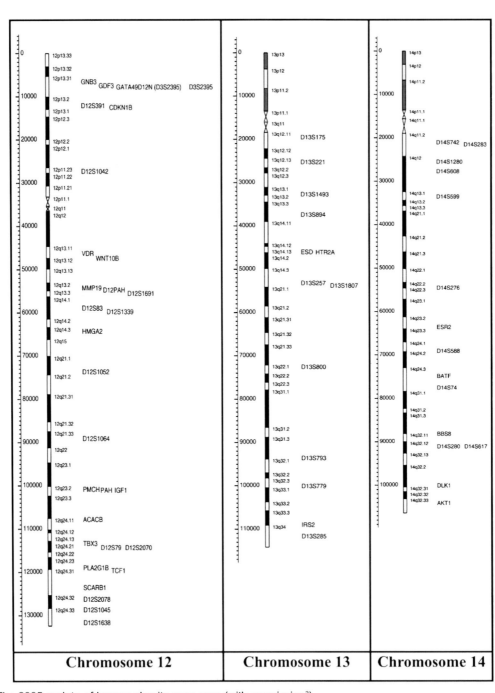

2.6 (*continued*) The 2005 update of human obesity gene map (with permission[3]).

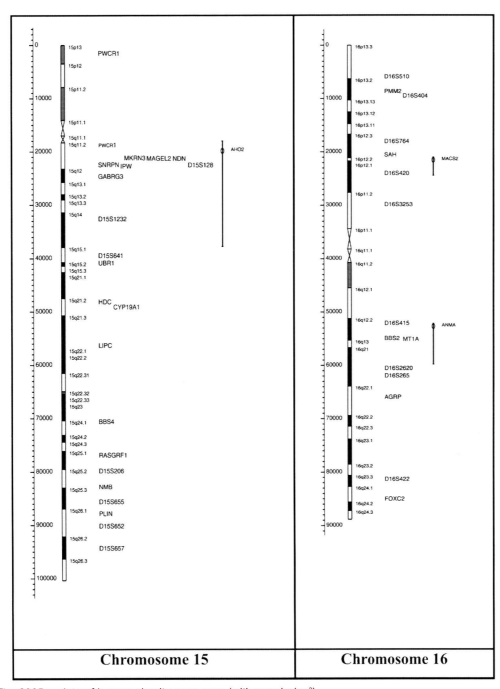

Chromosome 15   **Chromosome 16**

2.6 (*continued*) The 2005 update of human obesity gene map (with permission[3]).

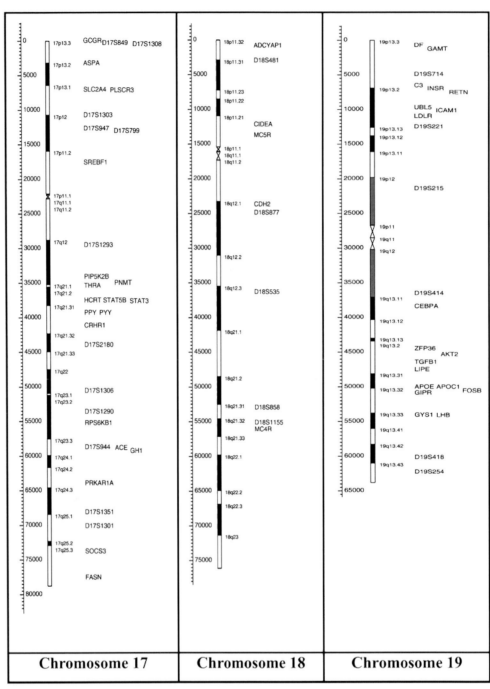

2.6 (*continued*) The 2005 update of human obesity gene map (with permission[3]).

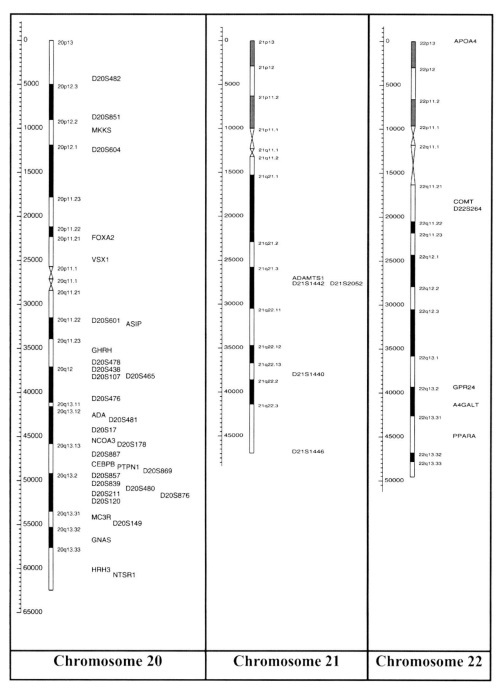

2.6 (*continued*) The 2005 update of human obesity gene map (with permission[3]).

Table 2.2 Genetic disorders associated with obesity

- Prader–Willi syndrome
- Laurence–Moon–Bardet–Biedl syndrome
- Down syndrome
- Congenital leptin deficiency
- Leptin resistance and leptin receptor mutations
- Proopiomelanocortin defects
- Melanocortin-4 receptor defects
- Albright hereditary osteodystrophy
- Alstrom–Hallgren syndrome
- Cohen syndrome
- Carpenter syndrome
- Grebe syndrome
- Beckwith–Wiedemann syndrome
- Adiposo-genital dystrophy syndrome
- Kleine–Levin–Critchley syndrome
- Young–Hughes syndrome
- Laron dwarfism
- X-linked mental retardation–hypotonic facies syndrome
- Borjeson–Forssman–Lehmann syndrome
- Pseudohypoparathyroidism type 1a
- Pro-hormone convertase 1 deficiency
- Neurotropin receptor (TrkB) deficiency

Fetal and infant origins of obesity

It has always been suspected that obesity and many other chronic diseases in adult life may be related to impaired fetal and infant growth. Numerous animal studies and some recent human observational studies have provided compelling evidence that the quantity and distribution of adipose tissue may be influenced during intrauterine and early postnatal life. A high body mass index during childhood and adolescence has been shown to predict adult obesity in longitudinal studies. For both obese and non-obese children less than 10 years of age, having an obese parent doubled the risk of becoming overweight in later life. There is evidence that weight at birth also correlates to adult weight.[8] Although increasing birth weight correlated with increased risk of adult obesity, it was noticed that people with the lowest birth weight (under 5.5 lbs) also had increased obesity prevalence. In particular, low birth weight is shown to be associated with increased truncal fat distribution.[8]

The rate of growth in early childhood also has an impact on subsequent levels of obesity. Babies who were born the smallest and then 'caught up fastest' were more likely to be obese in later life.

Fetal undernutrition and overnutrition are both thought to influence adult fat deposition and distribution. Socioeconomic status during early childhood is also shown to be a predictor of adult fatness. Possible explanations include the effects of infant and childhood feeding, undernourishment in early life followed by relative overnourishment, emotional deprivation leading to comfort eating later in life, and the tendency to follow cultural and social habits learnt during childhood. Maternal smoking is also thought to cause lower birth weight but a higher risk of obesity in adult life.

There is continuing debate about the role of infant feeding (in particular breast-feeding) and its relationship with adult obesity. Breast-feeding is thought to have a protective effect but the underlying mechanisms are not entirely clear. A meta-analysis of several large observational studies reported that a longer duration of breast-feeding is associated with a reduced risk of obesity in later life.[9]

Lifestyle and environmental factors influencing obesity

Environmental and behavioural changes in modern society have been blamed for the current world-wide increase in obesity, as the genetic and metabolic influences on an individual's susceptibility to obesity and the gene pool of the population as a whole have remained constant. Ethnic variations in susceptibility to obesity and population migration cannot explain the obesity epidemic. In fact, data from migration studies of some ethnic populations from developing countries have shown that the obesity risk increases dramatically when they are exposed to 'Western' lifestyles.

There has been no increase in the calories we eat per day in recent decades. The data from the UK National Food Survey (NFS) show that the average daily food intake in Britain has not changed significantly, but levels of physical activity have fallen.[10] However, there has been an increase in high-calorie (energy-dense) food intake and a fall in household food consumption. There has been a profound increase in the proportion of dietary fat consumption at the expense of carbohydrate intake[10] and there appears to be a strong correlation between dietary fat consumption and obesity risk.[11] Experimental studies show that consumption of energy-dense foods high in fat and sugar, produce a less powerful satiety response than foods high in complex carbohydrates, leading to the phenomenon of passive overconsumption. Moreover, studies that estimate food consumption are greatly confounded by under-reporting by obese subjects.

The levels of physical activity have dropped significantly over the last 50 years. The availability of labour-saving devices, better transportation facilities, changes in work patterns and the physical environment, lack of outdoor activity facilities, and sedentary leisure-time pursuits such as watching television and playing computer games have all been implicated in declining physical activity levels. There are some observational data to support the theory that time spent viewing television, particularly in children, and the availability and use of cars, are linked to an increase in obesity risk (**2.7–2.10**).[12]

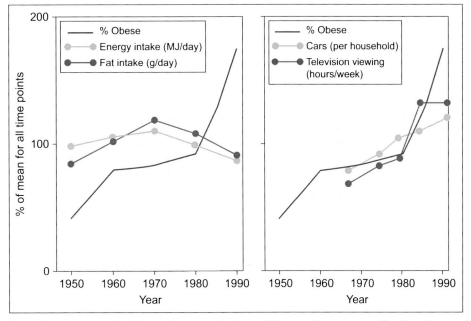

2.7 Secular trends in diet (left) and activity (right) in relation to obesity in Britain (with permission[10]). (Data for diet from National Food Survey; data for body mass index from Office of Population Censuses and Surveys and historical surveys; data for television viewing and car ownership from Central Statistical Office).

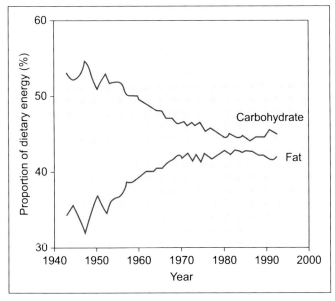

2.8 Changes in the fat/carbohydrate ratio of the British diet (source: National Food Survey) (with permission[10]).

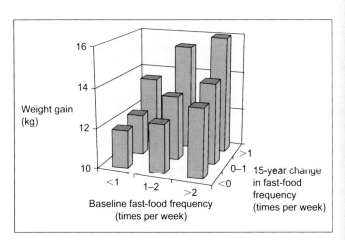

2.9 Fast food frequency over 15 years and weight gain (with permission[13]).

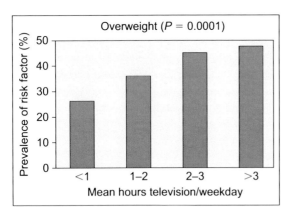

2.10 TV viewing time and the prevalence of obesity (with permission[12]).

Sleep deprivation is an under-reported lifestyle change that seems to have negative metabolic consequences. In one study, sleep restriction was associated with a decrease in serum leptin, increase in serum ghrelin, and increased hunger and appetite.[14] Inadequate sleep could lead to excessive eating and weight gain but currently there are only limited observational data to support this theory. Smoking cessation is often associated with an average weight gain of 4–5 kg. It is, therefore, important to offer dietary and exercise advice to people who are planning to quit smoking.

Successful management of an individual with obesity depends on a thorough assessment of his or her lifestyle. Detailed knowledge of eating patterns, food choices, work and social networks that influence dietary habits, frequency of eating, overall dietary fat intake, reliance on convenience foods, psychosocial factors, and the presence of eating disorders are essential before choosing an appropriate intervention. Similarly, lifestyle factors that limit physical activity and suggestions to improve daily energy expenditure are vital to the success of any therapy.

Secondary causes of obesity

Endocrine disease
Hypothyroidism, Cushing's syndrome, acromegaly, growth hormone deficiency, hypogonadism, and polycystic ovarian syndrome (PCOS) are all rare causes of weight gain. They are usually diagnosed before causing significant weight gain due the presence of multiple signs and symptoms. Ruling out these conditions is an important part of the assessment of a subject presenting with obesity.

Hypothalamic obesity
Tumours in the hypothalamic region, particularly craniopharyngiomas and pituitary macroadenomas with suprasellar extension, can damage the ventromedial hypothalamic areas that regulate energy intake (appetite regulation) and expenditure (**2.11**). This can also be caused by trauma, surgery, and radiation. These subjects can exhibit marked hyperphagia and have autonomic imbalance leading to hyperinsulinaemia, which can exacerbate weight gain by promoting fat deposition. Associated pituitary hormone imbalances and somnolence leading to reduced physical activity may contribute to their metabolic risk.

Drugs
Many drugs promote weight gain due to central effects on appetite and/or peripheral metabolic actions. Patients who are already overweight or at a risk of weight gain need to be aware of the side effects of the drugs that they take. Alternatives should be considered wherever possible or adequate measures must be taken to prevent weight gain. Some commonly used drugs associated with weight gain are listed in *Table 2.3*.

Pregnancy, contraception, and menopause
Weight gain during pregnancy is often significant in the history of women and there appears to be increased tendency to gain weight after pregnancy when compared with nulliparous women. Hormonal contraception has often been blamed for weight gain but the available evidence is not convincing. The decline in oestrogen and progesterone secretion after menopause seems to cause an alteration in adipocyte biology leading to weight gain and in particular an increase in central

Table 2.3 Drugs associated with weight gain

- Anticonvulsants
- Antipsychotics
- Antidepressants
- β-blockers
- Antihistamines
- Steroids
- Oral hypoglycaemic agents (except metformin and dipeptidyl peptidase 4 inhibitors)
- Insulin
- Protease inhibitors
- Sex hormones and contraceptive hormone preparations

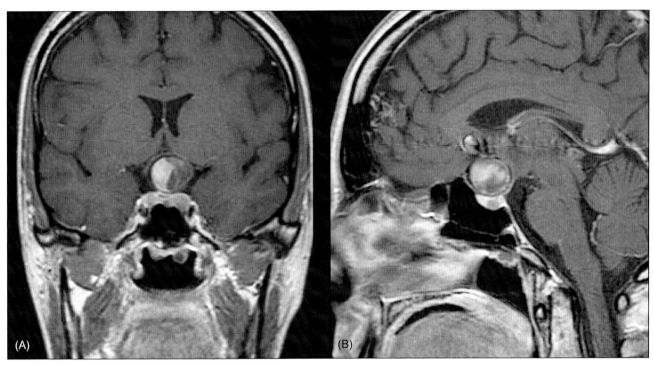

2.11 Tumours in the hypothalamic region shown by (A) coronal and (B) sagittal magnetic resonance imaging. Their treatment with surgery or radiotherapy is a common cause of hypothalamic obesity.

fat deposition. This is thought to be an important factor in increased cardiovascular risk after menopause.

Novel (unproven) theories

Intestinal flora

There have been some animal and human studies that propose a link between gut flora and obesity.[15] Intestinal flora in obese mice and humans are rich in firmicutes species and relatively deficient in bacteroides. Transplantation of gut flora from obese mice to lean mice promoted weight gain. In obese humans who lose weight, the gut flora changes to lean-type. These may be primary or secondary to changes in weight, or diet, or both.[15] Further studies are awaited before considering this as a significant factor in the pathophysiology of obesity.

Viral agents

Some infectious agents such as adenovirus have been implicated in the aetiology of obesity in animal studies. In one human study, the presence of adenovirus (AD-36) was associated with a higher body mass index, but lower cholesterol and triglyceride levels.[16]

References

1. Neary NM, Goldstone AP, Bloom SR. Appetite regulation: from the gut to the hypothalamus. *Clin Endocrinol (Oxf)* 2004; **60**: 153–60.
2. Farooqi IS, Jebb SA, Langmack G, *et al.* Effects of recombinant leptin therapy in a child with congenital leptin deficiency. *N Engl J Med* 1999; **341**: 879–84.
3. Rankinen T, Zuberi A, Chagnon YC, *et al.* The human obesity gene map: the 2005 update. *Obesity (Silver Spring)* 2006; **14**: 529–644.
4. Farooqi IS. Monogenic human obesity. *Front Horm Res* 2008; **36**: 1–11.
5. Frayling TM, Timpson NJ, Weedon MN, *et al.* A common variant in the FTO gene is associated with body mass index and predisposes to childhood and adult obesity. *Science* 2007; **316**: 889–94.
6. Loos RJ, Bouchard C. FTO: the first gene contributing to common forms of human obesity. *Obes Rev* 2008; **9**: 246–50.
7. Herbert A, Gerry NP, McQueen MB, *et al.* A common genetic variant is associated with adult and childhood obesity. *Science* 2006; **312**: 279–83.

8. Barker M, Robinson S, Osmond C, Barker DJ. Birth weight and body fat distribution in adolescent girls. *Arch Dis Child* 1997; **77**: 381–3.

9. Harder T, Bergmann R, Kallischnigg G, Plagemann A. Duration of breastfeeding and risk of overweight: a meta-analysis. *Am J Epidemiol* 2005; **162**: 397–403.

10. Prentice AM, Jebb SA. Obesity in Britain: gluttony or sloth? *BMJ* 1995; **311**: 437–9.

11. Lissner L, Heitmann BL. Dietary fat and obesity: evidence from epidemiology. *Eur J Clin Nutr* 1995; **49**: 79–90.

12. Hancox RJ, Milne BJ, Poulton R. Association between child and adolescent television viewing and adult health: a longitudinal birth cohort study. *Lancet* 2004; **364**: 257–62.

13. Pereira MA, Kartashov AI, Ebbeling CB, *et al.* Fast-food habits, weight gain, and insulin resistance (the CARDIA study): 15-year prospective analysis. *Lancet* 2005; **365**: 36–42.

14. Spiegel K, Tasali E, Penev P, Van CE. Brief communication: sleep curtailment in healthy young men is associated with decreased leptin levels, elevated ghrelin levels, and increased hunger and appetite. *Ann Intern Med* 2004; **141**: 846–50.

15. Ley RE, Turnbaugh PJ, Klein S, Gordon JI. Microbial ecology: human gut microbes associated with obesity. *Nature* 2006; **444**: 1022–3.

16. Atkinson RL, Dhurandhar NV, Allison DB, *et al.* Human adenovirus-36 is associated with increased body weight and paradoxical reduction of serum lipids. *Int J Obes (Lond)* 2005; **29**: 281–6.

Associations and complications of obesity

The associations and complications of obesity in adults, and in children and adolescents are summarized in *Tables 3.1* and *3.2*.

Table 3.1 Associations and complications in adults

Metabolic associations	Metabolic syndrome Insulin resistance, type 2 diabetes Impaired glucose tolerance Impaired fasting glucose Dyslipidaemia Prothrombotic and pro-inflammatory state
Cardiovascular	Sudden death Vascular disease: ischaemic heart disease, cerebrovascular disease, peripheral vascular disease Hypertension Cardiomyopathy Congestive cardiac failure, cor pulmonale Arrhythmias
Respiratory	Obstructive sleep apnoea Asthma Obesity hypoventilation syndrome Restrictive lung disease Pulmonary embolism
Gastrointestinal	Fatty liver, steatohepatitis Gastro-oesophageal reflux disease Gallstones, cholecystitis Altered bowel habits
Cancer	Breast Colorectal, oesophageal Endometrial Kidney, prostate
Fertility and genitourinary	Subfertility Polycystic ovary syndrome Erectile dysfunction Pregnancy related complications, fetal defects Urinary incontinence Renal impairment, obesity-related glomerulopathy Kidney stones
Musculoskeletal	Osteoarthritis Gout and hyperuricaemia
Psychosocial	Depression, low self-esteem Daytime sleepiness, fatigue Body dysmorphic disorder Social stigmatization Absenteeism Impaired quality of life
Neurological	Stroke Autonomic dysfunction Headaches, migraine Dementia Parkinson's disease Benign intracranial hypertension Carpal tunnel
Miscellaneous	Increased anaesthetic and surgical risk Varicose veins, deep venous thrombosis Lymphoedema Cataract Hernia Skin complications, cellulitis

Table 3.2 Associations and complications in children and adolescents

General	Adult obesity Increased adult mortality and morbidity	Orthopaedic	Foot pronation, flat feet Tibia vara (Blount's disease) Slipped capital femoral epiphysis Tibial torsion Ankle sprains, increased risk of fractures
Cardiovascular	Hypertension Cardiac muscle abnormalities: left ventricular hypertrophy Fatty streaks Abnormal blood vessel structure and function Increased heart rate variability	Gastrointestinal	Hepatic steatosis Gastro-oesophageal reflux Cholelithiasis
		Neurological	Benign intracranial hypertension
		Psychosocial	Lowered self-worth Body dissatisfaction Reduced cognitive function Behavioural disorders Depression and anxiety Substance abuse Restricted social networks Disordered eating
Respiratory	Sleep: disordered breathing Pickwickian syndrome Asthma		
Metabolic and endocrine	Metabolic syndrome Insulin resistance, type 2 diabetes Impaired glucose tolerance Hyperlipidaemia Acanthosis nigricans Changed onset of puberty Menstrual abnormalities Polycystic ovaries Hypercorticism Systemic inflammation Raised C-reactive protein	Minor consequences	Heat intolerance Heat rash, intertrigo, and furunculosis Breathlessness on exertion Tiredness Musculoskeletal discomfort Pseudogynaecomastia Male genitalia of small appearance Cutaneous striae

Metabolic syndrome: diabetes, dyslipidaemia, and insulin resistance

Metabolic syndrome is characterized by a cluster of medical disorders that often occur together in one individual, which increases the risk of cardiovascular disease and diabetes. Several definitions and criteria exist but the important components and associations that are thought to represent metabolic syndrome are summarized in *Tables 3.3–3.8*.

In 1998, the American Diabetes Association (ADA) issued a consensus statement identifying 'glucose intolerance, central obesity, dyslipidaemia (increased triglycerides, decreased high-density lipoprotein, increased small dense low-density lipoprotein), hypertension, increased prothrombotic and antifibrinolytic factors, and a predilection for atherosclerotic vascular disease' as components of the metabolic syndrome associated with insulin resistance. The American Diabetes Association statement did not provide diagnostic cut-points or criteria for the syndrome.

Obesity is strongly and independently linked to all the other components of metabolic syndrome described in *Table 3.3*. The Third Report of the National Cholesterol Education Program (NCEP-ATP III) and American Heart Association/National Heart, Lung and Blood Institute (AHA/NHLBI) guidelines did not include abdominal obesity as a requirement for diagnosis because lesser degrees of abdominal girth are often associated with other components. However, the International Diabetes Federation (IDF) consensus statement includes central obesity as a prerequisite for diagnosis.

Table 3.3 Metabolic syndrome: proposed components and associated findings[1]

1. Insulin resistance*
2. Hyperinsulinaemia*
3. Obesity: visceral (central), but also generalized obesity*
4. Dyslipidaemia: high triglycerides, low high-density lipoprotein, small dense low-density lipoprotein*
5. Adipocyte dysfunction
6. Impaired glucose tolerance or type 2 diabetes mellitus*
7. Fatty liver (non-alcoholic steatohepatosis, steatohepatitis)
8. Essential hypertension: increased systolic and diastolic blood pressure*
9. Endothelial dysfunction
10. Renal dysfunction: micro- or macroalbuminuria
11. Polycystic ovary syndrome
12. Inflammation: increased C-reactive protein and other inflammatory markers
13. Hypercoagulability: increased fibrinogen and plasminogen activating inhibitor 1
14. Atherosclerosis leading to increased cardiovascular morbidity and mortality*

*Most widely incorporated into the definition of metabolic syndrome.

Table 3.4 WHO definition of metabolic syndrome[2]

Impaired glucose tolerance, impaired fasting glucose, diabetes and/or insulin resistance (defined as highest quartile of $HOMA_{IR}$) and ≥ 2 of the following:

Obesity	
BMI	>30 kg/m² or
Waist-to-hip ratio	>0.85 women, >0.90 men
Dyslipidaemia	
Triglycerides	≥ 1.7 mmol/l (≥ 150 mg/dl) or
High-density lipoprotein	<0.9 mmol/l (<35 mg/dl) in men
	<1.0 mmol/l (<39 mg/dl) women
Blood pressure	$\geq 140/90$ mmHg
Microalbuminuria	
Urinary excretion rate	≥ 20 µg/min or
Albumin–creatinine ratio	≥ 20 mg/g

Table 3.5 Diagnosis of metabolic syndrome suggested by the National Cholesterol Education Program (NCEP-ATP III)[3]

Presence of ≥3 of the following risk factors:

Abdominal obesity (waist circumference)

Men	>102 cm (>40 inches)
Women	>88 cm (>35 inches)

Triglycerides	≥1.7 mmol/l (≥150 mg/dl)

High-density lipoprotein

Men	<1.04 mmol/l (<40 mg/dl)
Women	<1.3 mmol/l (<50 mg/dl)
Blood pressure	≥130/≥85 mmHg
Fasting glucose	≥6.1 mmol/l (≥110 mg/dl)

Table 3.6 The new International Diabetes Federation definition of metabolic syndrome[4]

Central obesity – defined by waist circumference (see Table 3.7 for ethnicity specific values) with any two of the following four factors:

Raised triglycerides	≥150 mg/dl (≥1.7 mmol/l) or specific treatment for this lipid abnormality
Reduced high-density lipoprotein cholesterol	<40 mg/dl (1.03 mmol/l) in men <50 mg/dl (1.29 mmol/l) in women or specific treatment for this lipid abnormality
Raised BP	Systolic BP ≥130 or diastolic BP ≥85 mmHg or treatment of previously diagnosed hypertension
Raised FPG	FPG ≥100 mg/dl (≥5.6 mmol/l) or previously diagnosed type 2 diabetes. If above 5.6 mmol/l or 100 mg/dl, OGTT is strongly recommended but is not necessary to define presence of the syndrome.

If BMI is >30 kg/m^2, central obesity can be assumed and waist circumference does not need to be measured.
BP, blood pressure; FPG, fasting plasma glucose; OGTT, oral glucose tolerance test.

Most of the above definitions recognize central obesity [categorized by waist circumference or waist-to-hip ratio (WHR)] as the essential component of metabolic syndrome rather than generalized obesity, as the intra-abdominal fat content has a stronger correlation with insulin resistance and hyperinsulinaemia. The relationship between insulin resistance and cardiovascular disease was described by Reaven (**3.1**).[6]

Epidemiological data show that the increase in prevalence of obesity closely mirrors increases in the prevalence of type 2 diabetes. The pathophysiological links between obesity, type 2 diabetes, and metabolic syndrome are well established (**3.2–3.7**).[7]

Obesity is strongly linked to dyslipidaemia (**3.8**), which is almost always included in the diagnostic criteria for metabolic

Table 3.7 Ethnic specific values for waist circumference. Central obesity is most easily measured by waist circumference using the guidelines in the table, which are gender and ethnic group (not country of residence) specific

Country/ethnic group	Waist circumference
Europids* In the USA, the ATP III values (102 cm men; 88 cm women) are likely to continue to be used for clinical purposes	Male ≥94 cm Female ≥80 cm
South Asians Based on a Chinese, Malay and Asian-Indian population	Male ≥90 cm Female ≥80 cm
Chinese	Male ≥90 cm Female ≥80 cm
Japanese†	Male ≥90 cm Female ≥80 cm
Ethnic South and Central Americans	Use South Asian recommendations until more specific data are available
Sub-Saharan Africans	Use European data until more specific data are available
Eastern Mediterranean and Middle East (Arab) populations	Use European data until more specific data are available

*In future epidemiological studies of populations of Europid origin, prevalence should be given using both European and North American cut-points to allow better comparisons.
†Originally, different values were proposed for Japanese people, but new data support the use of the values shown above.

Table 3.8 American Heart Association/National Heart, Lung and Blood Institute (AHA/NHLBI) criteria[5]

Presence of any three of the following:

Elevated waist circumference	
Men	≥102 cm (40 inches)
Women	≥88 cm (35 inches)
Elevated triglycerides	≥1.7 mmol/l (150 mg/dl) or on drug treatment (e.g. fibrates, nicotinic acid)
Reduced high-density lipoprotein cholesterol	
Men	<1.03 mmol/l (<40 mg/dl)
Women	<1.3 mmol/l (<50 mg/dl)
Elevated blood pressure	≥130/≥85 mmHg or on medication for hypertension
Elevated fasting glucose	≥100 mg/dl (≥5.6 mmol/l) or on medication for hyperglycaemia

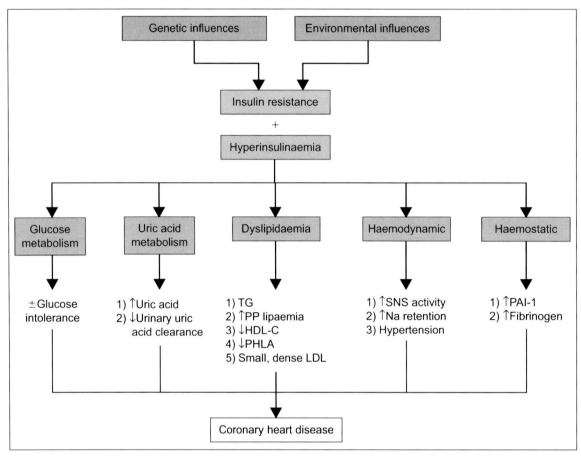

3.1 Relationship between insulin resistance and coronary heart disease (with permission[6]). HDL-C, high-density lipoprotein cholesterol; LDL, low-density lipoprotein; PAI-1, plasminogen activator inhibitor-1; PHLA, post-heparin lipolytic activity; PP, post prandial; SNS, sympathetic nervous system; TG, triglyceride.

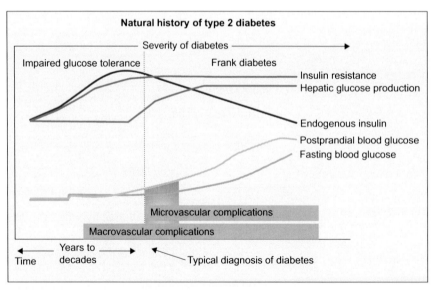

3.2 Pathophysiology of metabolic syndrome components and type 2 diabetes (with permission[7]).

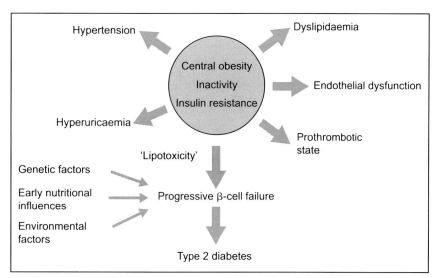

3.3 Relationship between the major components of metabolic syndrome and type 2 diabetes (with permission[25])

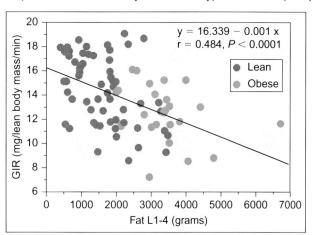

3.4 Relationship between central obesity and insulin resistance. Graph shows the relationship between glucose infusion rate (GIR) (mg/kg lean body mass/min) and fat mass at level L1–4 in lean and obese subjects (with permission[8]).

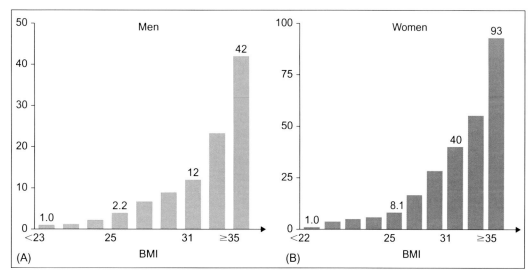

3.5 Age-adjusted relative risk of developing type 2 diabetes according to BMI: (A) men (with permission[9]); (B) women (with permission[10]).

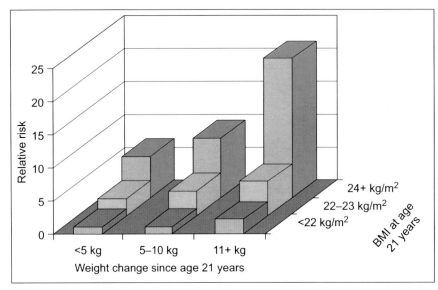

3.6 Weight gain in adult life as a predictor of diabetes (with permission[9]).

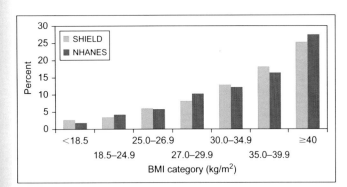

3.7 Prevalence of diabetes mellitus by BMI level (with permission[11,12]) (data from: (1) Study to Help Improve Early evaluation and management of risk factors Leading to Diabetes (SHIELD), and (2) National Health and Nutrition Examination Surveys (NHANES)).

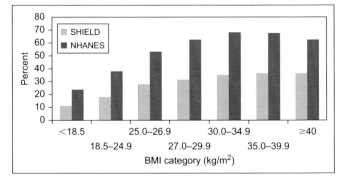

3.8 Prevalence of dyslipidaemia by BMI level (with permission[11,12]) (data from: (1) Study to Help Improve Early evaluation and management of risk factors Leading to Diabetes (SHIELD), and (2) National Health and Nutrition Examination Surveys (NHANES)).

syndrome. The 'lipid overflow–ectopic fat model' or the 'hypertriglyceridic waist' model proposes that disturbances in lipid metabolism play a vital role in the pathogenesis of metabolic syndrome (**3.9**).[13]

It is now well established that the amount of visceral obesity is more closely linked to metabolic complications than generalized obesity. In order to understand the relative contributions of total body fatness and visceral adipose tissue, the metabolic parameters were compared between two groups of obese men with the same amount of total body fat, but with either low or high levels of visceral adipose tissue. The plasma triglyceride and high-density lipoprotein levels between these two groups and

lean controls were compared (**3.10**).[14] In addition to these changes, obese men with high visceral adipose tissue had significantly higher levels of fasting plasma insulin and a higher insulin and glucose response to a standard oral glucose load (**3.11**).[14]

Cardiovascular

Obesity is strongly associated with several known cardiovascular risk factors such as hypertension, type 2 diabetes, and dyslipidaemia, and is also recognized as an independent risk factor for cardiovascular mortality and

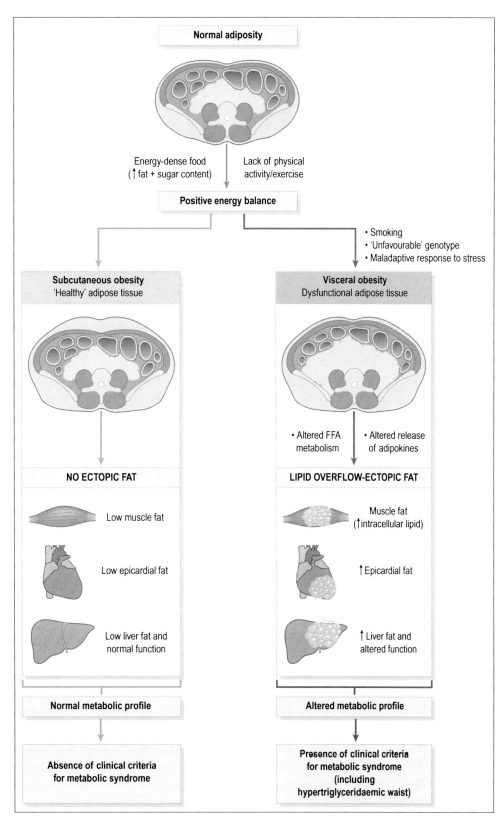

3.9 In addition to total fat mass, unfavourable fat distribution also determines the risk of metabolic syndrome and its associated complications. This figure demonstrates the likely link between disturbances in lipid metabolism and metabolic syndrome (with permission[13]).

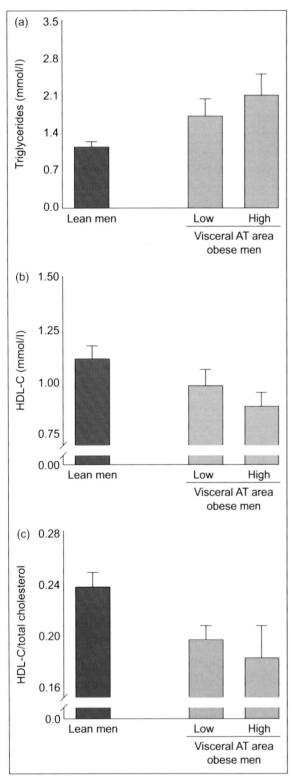

3.10 Charts showing the comparison of (A) triglycerides, (B) HDL, and (C) HDL-C/total cholesterol ratio in lean, obese + low visceral fat and obese + high visceral fat men (with permission[14]). AT, adipose tissue; HDL, high-density lipoprotein; HDL-C, HDL cholesterol.

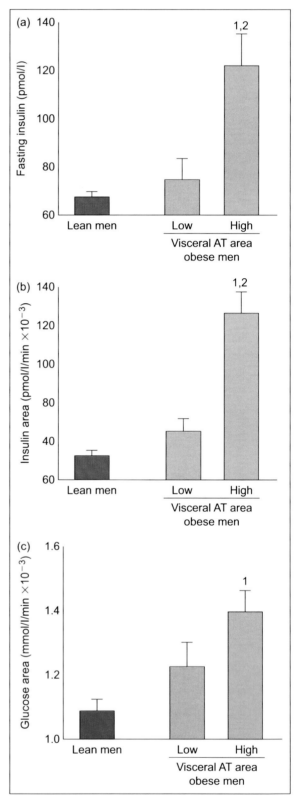

3.11 (A) Fasting insulin levels, (B) insulin, and (C) glucose response to standard oral glucose load in lean, obese + low visceral fat, and obese + high visceral fat men (with permission[14]).

morbidity (**3.12**). Most, but not all, obese individuals also have impaired cardiovascular 'fitness', which predicts increased mortality from cardiovascular disease independently of the degree of obesity.

Sudden death

Obesity increases the risk of sudden death, probably by a variety of mechanisms, including increased sympathetic nerve activity, prolongation of the QT interval, and structural heart disease such as coronary heart disease (CHD) and cardiomyopathy (**3.13**). The strong association between obesity and obstructive sleep apnoea (OSA) is also likely to contribute to the increased risk of sudden death.

Vascular disease

In a prospective cohort study of 44 702 US female registered nurses aged between 40 and 65 years, measurements of both central and total obesity were independently associated with an increased risk of CHD in stratified analyses. As shown in **3.14**, a higher WHR was associated with increased age-adjusted risk of CHD, regardless of body mass index (BMI) tertile. Within any BMI tertile, women in the highest WHR tertile had a twofold higher incidence of CHD than in the lowest WHR tertile. Within each WHR tertile, higher BMI also was generally associated with increased risk. As shown in **3.15**, within each tertile of BMI, larger waist circumference was also associated with increased risk of CHD.[16]

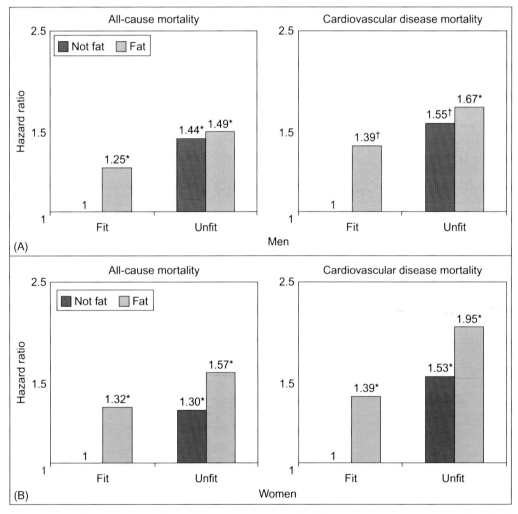

3.12 Adjusted mortality hazard for fatness and fitness in men and women. (A) Relative hazard in men categorized by fitness level (quintile 1 vs quintiles 2–5) and BMI (quintiles 1–4 vs quintile 5) adjusted for age, education, smoking, alcohol, and Keys score. (B) Relative hazard in women categorized by fitness level (quintile 1 vs quintiles 2–5) and BMI (quintiles 1–4 vs quintile 5) adjusted for age, education, smoking, alcohol, and Keys score (with permission[15]). * = P <0.05; † = P <0.06.

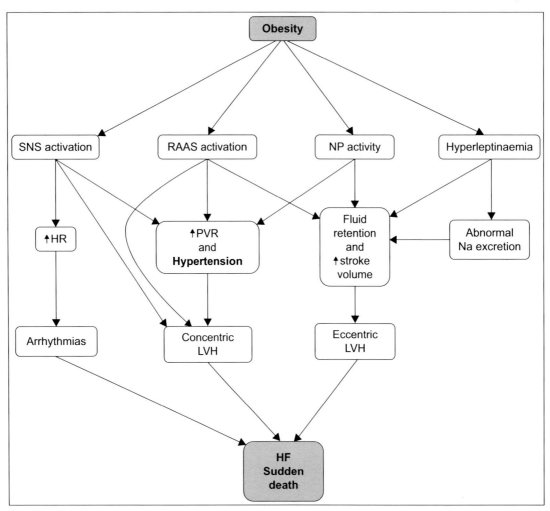

3.13 A summary of the mechanisms by which obesity may lead to excessive cardiovascular morbidity and mortality (with permission[17]). ↑, increase; BP, blood pressure; HF, heart failure; HR, heart rate; LVH, left ventricular hypertrophy; Na, sodium; NP, natriuretic peptide; PVR, peripheral vascular resistance; RAAS, renin–angiotensin–aldosterone system; SNS, sympathetic nervous system.

The INTERHEART study was a case–control study involving 29 972 participants in 52 countries. The study examined the contribution of various cardiometabolic risk factors to the risk of a first acute myocardial infarction (AMI). It quantified the relationships between risk factors and AMI through calculation of the population attributable risk (PAR), which measures the proportion of AMI among those who have the risk factor that would be eliminated if the risk factor was removed (**3.16A**). Dyslipidaemia (raised apolipoprotein B/A1 ratio) and smoking were associated with the highest PAR. However, PAR for abdominal obesity was greater than either diabetes or hypertension (**3.16B**). BMI showed a modest correlation with the risk of AMI, but this was not significant when abdominal obesity was included in a multivariate analysis.

Abdominal obesity is therefore an important predictor of adverse cardiovascular outcomes in its own right.

Role of visceral fat in inflammation

Visceral fat is an active endocrine organ producing a number of factors (adipokines) that may contribute to local and systemic inflammation in obesity (**3.17**). Some of these factors are also involved directly and indirectly in the control of vascular tone, endothelial function, coagulation, and insulin sensitivity. Local production and circulatory concentrations of most adipokines are increased in obesity, although adiponectin (generally considered as a protective factor) decreases as BMI rises. Increased levels of tumour necrosis factor-α and interleukin-6 may promote insulin resistance in obesity, whereas adiponectin reduces insulin

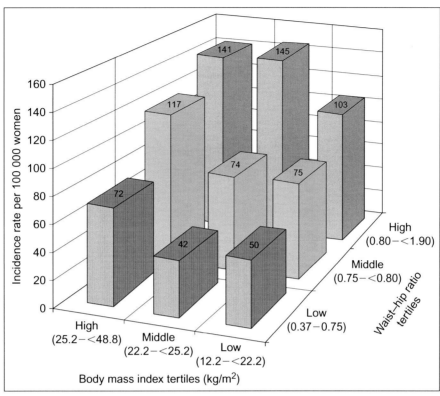

3.14 Age-adjusted incidence rates for coronary heart disease according to BMI and waist–hip ratio tertiles (with permission[16]). Numbers at the top of each bar indicate incidence.

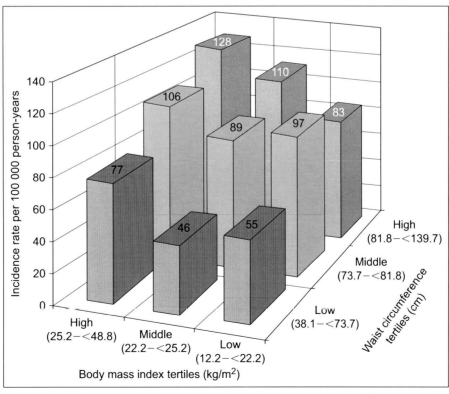

3.15 Age-adjusted incidence rates for coronary heart disease according to BMI and waist circumference tertiles (with permission[16]).

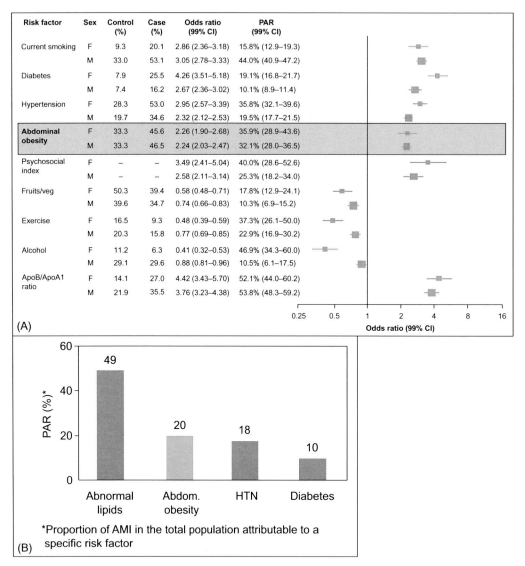

Risk factor	Sex	Control (%)	Case (%)	Odds ratio (99% CI)	PAR (99% CI)
Current smoking	F	9.3	20.1	2.86 (2.36–3.18)	15.8% (12.9–19.3)
	M	33.0	53.1	3.05 (2.78–3.33)	44.0% (40.9–47.2)
Diabetes	F	7.9	25.5	4.26 (3.51–5.18)	19.1% (16.8–21.7)
	M	7.4	16.2	2.67 (2.36–3.02)	10.1% (8.9–11.4)
Hypertension	F	28.3	53.0	2.95 (2.57–3.39)	35.8% (32.1–39.6)
	M	19.7	34.6	2.32 (2.12–2.53)	19.5% (17.7–21.5)
Abdominal obesity	F	33.3	45.6	2.26 (1.90–2.68)	35.9% (28.9–43.6)
	M	33.3	46.5	2.24 (2.03–2.47)	32.1% (28.0–36.5)
Psychosocial index	F	–	–	3.49 (2.41–5.04)	40.0% (28.6–52.6)
	M	–	–	2.58 (2.11–3.14)	25.3% (18.2–34.0)
Fruits/veg	F	50.3	39.4	0.58 (0.48–0.71)	17.8% (12.9–24.1)
	M	39.6	34.7	0.74 (0.66–0.83)	10.3% (6.9–15.2)
Exercise	F	16.5	9.3	0.48 (0.39–0.59)	37.3% (26.1–50.0)
	M	20.3	15.8	0.77 (0.69–0.85)	22.9% (16.9–30.2)
Alcohol	F	11.2	6.3	0.41 (0.32–0.53)	46.9% (34.3–60.0)
	M	29.1	29.6	0.88 (0.81–0.96)	10.5% (6.1–17.5)
ApoB/ApoA1 ratio	F	14.1	27.0	4.42 (3.43–5.70)	52.1% (44.0–60.2)
	M	21.9	35.5	3.76 (3.23–4.38)	53.8% (48.3–59.2)

Odds ratio (99% CI)

(A)

(B) *Proportion of AMI in the total population attributable to a specific risk factor

PAR (%)*
- Abnormal lipids: 49
- Abdom. obesity: 20
- HTN: 18
- Diabetes: 10

3.16 (A) Odds ratio for myocardial infarction showing how abdominal obesity more than doubles the odds of AMI. (B) Risk factors for myocardial infarction, showing how abdominal obesity predicts the risk of CVD beyond BMI (with permission[18]). AMI, acute myocardial infarction; Apo, apolipoprotein; BMI, body mass index; CI, confidence interval; CVD, cardiovascular disease; HTN, hypertension; PAR, population attributable risk.

resistance. Adipose tissue is also a source of plasminogen activator inhibitor-1, haptoglobin (which increases blood coagulability), and angiotensinogen (which raises blood pressure). Intercellular adhesion molecule-1 and retinol binding protein-4 may contribute via increased oxidative stress leading to endothelial dysfunction.

Hypertension and cardiac failure

The exact mechanism whereby obesity causes hypertension is still unknown. Several models have been proposed to explain how obesity influences blood pressure (*see* **3.26**).

Epidemiological data confirm that the risk of hypertension correlates with the degree of obesity (**3.18–3.20**).

Respiratory disease and obstructive sleep apnoea

As the prevalence of obesity increases, clinicians are seeing increasing numbers of patients with obesity-related lung disease (**3.21**). Breathlessness is a common respiratory symptom; in obesity, this may be brought on by deconditioning or increased

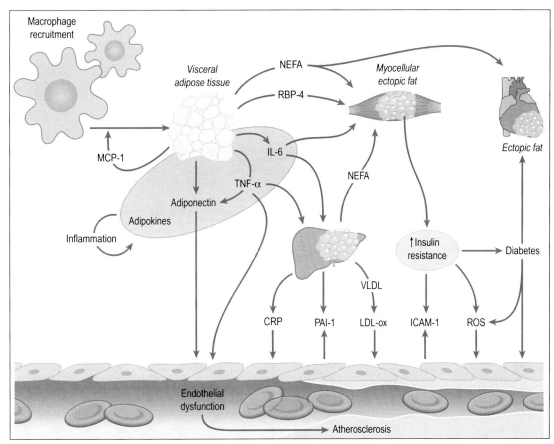

3.17 Visceral fat deposits and the associated insulin resistance contribute significantly to increased cardiovascular disease in obesity. Excess visceral fat leads to endothelial dysfunction and inflammation through the direct and indirect effects of adipokines (adiponectin and TNF-α). Fat accumulation, insulin resistance, liver-induced inflammation, and dyslipidaemia may all lead to the premature atherosclerotic process (with permission[19]). CRP, C-reactive protein; ICAM-1, intercellular adhesion molecule-1; IL-6, interleukin-6; LDL, low-density lipoprotein; LDL-ox, oxidised low-density lipoprotein; MCP-1, monocyte chemoattractant protein-1; NEFA, non-esterified fatty accids; PAI-1, plasminogen activator inhibitor-1; RBP-4, retinol-binding protein-4; ROS, reactive oxygen species; TNF-α, tumour necrosis factor-alpha; VLDL, very low-density lipoprotein.

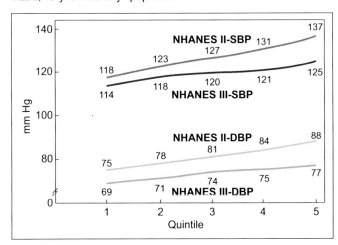

3.18 Line graph shows age-adjusted systolic blood pressure (SBP) and diastolic blood pressure (DBP) from the National Health and Nutrition Examination Surveys (NHANES) II and III by NHANES III quintile of BMI (source: Centers for Disease Control and Prevention (CDC), National Centers for Health Statistics).

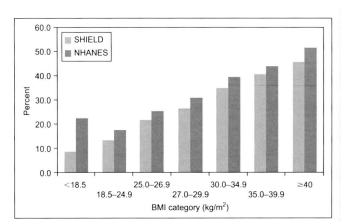

3.19 Prevalence of hypertension by BMI level (with permission[11,12]) (data from: (1) Study to Help Improve Early evaluation and management of risk factors Leading to Diabetes (SHIELD), and (2) National Health and Nutrition Examination Surveys (NHANES)).

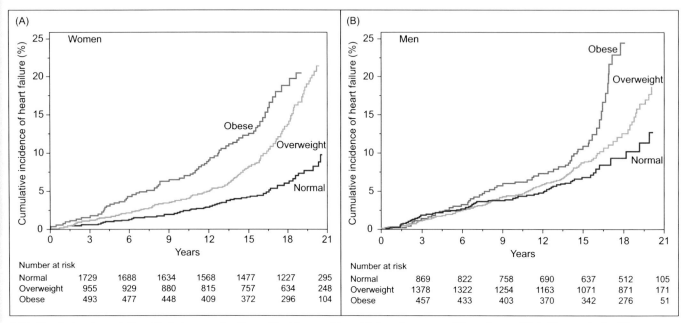

3.20 Chart showing relationship between obesity and incidence of heart failure in women (A) and men (B) (with permission[20]). Cumulative incidence of heart failure according to category of BMI at the baseline examination. The BMI was 18.5–24.9 in normal subjects, 25–29.9 in overweight subjects, and 30 or more in obese subjects.

work of breathing due to the excessive weight being carried, rather than lung disease itself. It is also important to consider that the breathlessness may arise from cardiovascular disease. However, there are a number of respiratory conditions that are linked to obesity.

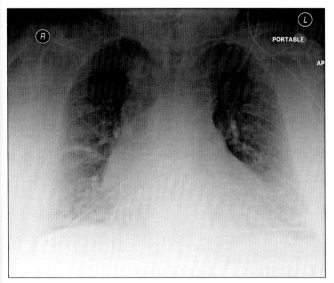

3.21 Chest X-ray of an obese patient showing cardiomegaly, congested lung fields, and restriction. This patient was known to suffer from cor pulmonale, obstructive sleep apnoea, and obesity hypoventilation requiring non-invasive ventilation.

Lung function

Cross-sectional and longitudinal studies have demonstrated that increases in body weight are linked to a reduction in lung function. As BMI increases, the forced expiratory volume in 1 second (FEV_1), forced vital capacity (FVC), total lung capacity, functional residual capacity, and expiratory reserve volume decrease, although these changes may not be evident until the BMI is >40 kg/m^2. Truncal obesity leads to direct mechanical effects by impeding movement of the diaphragm and chest wall and this may be reflected in a restrictive spirometry pattern (FEV_1/FVC ratio >0.7). Respiratory muscle strength may also be reduced in obesity (reduced chest wall compliance and operating lung volumes may lead to reduced muscle efficiency). Ventilation/perfusion abnormalities and arterial hypoxaemia at the lung bases also arise as a result of obesity.

Asthma

Asthma is defined by episodic airflow obstruction, increased airways responsiveness, and airways inflammation; common symptoms are cough, wheeze, and breathlessness. There is a clear link between obesity and a clinical diagnosis of asthma, although there is conflicting evidence as to whether airways hyper-responsiveness or allergy is increased by obesity. The incidence of asthma is increased by 50% in obese subjects.

In patients with pre-existing asthma, increased BMI is linked with worse asthma control. The relationships between asthma and obesity are complex.

- *Mechanical factors.* The impact of obesity on pulmonary function has been described above. The reduced operating lung volumes may compromise the dilating forces that maintain the patency of the airways, leading to airway resistance, which in turn causes airflow obstruction.
- *Inflammation.* Fat tissue produces several inflammatory mediators. Increased levels of these mediators in obese subjects may be linked with asthma or impaired asthma control.
- *Hormonal.* There appears to be a greater link between asthma and obesity in women than men. Obesity is linked to increased oestrogen levels, which may modulate the immune and inflammatory response.
- *Genetics and* in-utero *experience.* Certain genes that are associated with obesity are clustered in close proximity to those linked with asthma. A low birth weight is associated with an increased incidence of asthma later in life, while

other studies have linked both low and high birth weight to obesity. There are few data on the relationships between birth weight, obesity, and asthma.

A cornerstone of asthma treatment is corticosteroid therapy. While inhaled steroids very rarely result in weight gain, it is well known that prolonged oral steroid therapy increases appetite, leading to increased BMI, which may in turn further worsen the asthma.

Although the mechanisms behind the links between asthma and obesity are poorly understood, it is clear that there is a link and some studies have shown that weight loss results in better asthma control.

Obstructive sleep apnoea
OSA is a condition in which there is intermittent and repeated upper airway collapse during sleep. Pharyngeal muscles fail to maintain upper airway patency, resulting in intermittent upper airway obstruction. This leads to episodic hypoxaemia, hypercapnia, and blood pressure surges (**3.22**). Patients (or their bed partner) may report snoring, apnoeic spells

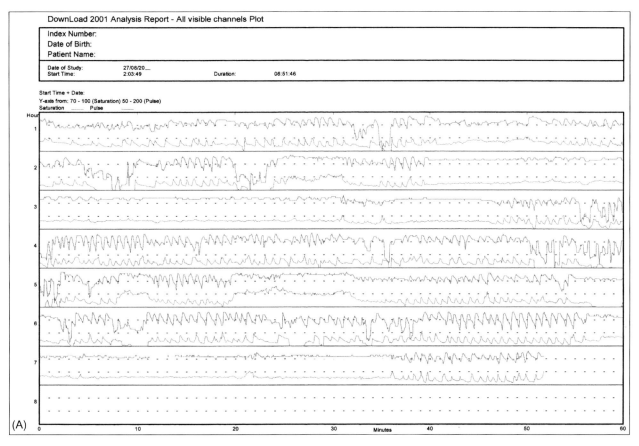

3.22 (A) An overnight oximetry trace showing significant desaturations and reflex tachycardias, highly suggestive of sleep apnoea.

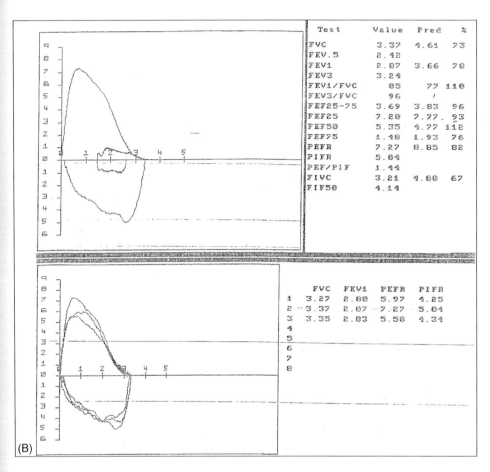

Test	Value	Pred	%
FVC	3.37	4.61	73
FEV.5	2.42		
FEV1	2.87	3.66	78
FEV3	3.24		
FEV1/FVC	85	77	110
FEV3/FVC	96	/	
FEF25-75	3.69	3.83	96
FEF25	7.28	7.77	93
FEF50	5.35	4.77	112
FEF75	1.48	1.93	76
PEFR	7.27	8.85	82
PIFR	5.04		
PEF/PIF	1.44		
FIVC	3.21	4.80	67
FIF50	4.14		

	FVC	FEV1	PEFR	PIFR
1	3.27	2.88	5.97	4.25
2	3.37	2.87	7.27	5.04
3	3.35	2.83	5.58	4.34
4				
5				
6				
7				
8				

(B)

3.22 (*continued*) (B) Flow-volume loop typical of morbid obesity.

and choking episodes at night. They may feel unrefreshed after sleep and report excessive daytime sleepiness (**3.23**). OSA is associated with increased mortality from accidents (particularly road traffic accidents) and cardiovascular disorders associated with this condition. Obesity is a major risk factor for OSA: up to 70% of patients with OSA are obese, and approximately 40% of obese patients have OSA. Reduced operating lung volumes, increased airway collapsibility and increased fat deposition in the soft tissues of the neck contribute to the development of OSA.

The prevalence of OSA is increasing in parallel with the increase in obesity. However, this condition is still under-recognized and under-reported. The condition is treatable, usually in the form of nasal continuous positive-airway pressure (CPAP) delivered overnight (**3.24**). In many cases, CPAP can be discontinued if the patient achieves significant weight loss.

Obesity hypoventilation syndrome

Obesity hypoventilation syndrome (OHS) is characterized by hypoxaemia, hypercapnia, and obesity in the absence of other causes for hypoventilation. It is estimated that one-fifth of patients with OSA also have obesity hypoventilation syndrome, although this syndrome is often missed in many patients. There is uncertainty about the exact mechanisms behind the development of this disorder: the restrictive lung mechanics associated with obesity play a role, along with a loss of respiratory drive. Interventions that may improve this condition include weight loss or nocturnal oxygen delivery, but in most cases, non-invasive overnight ventilatory support is required (CPAP or bi-level ventilation). Untreated, patients with obesity hypoventilation syndrome develop pulmonary hypertension and cardiac failure and mortality rates (usually from cardiorespiratory causes) are very high in these patients (**3.25**).

EPWORTH SLEEPINESS SCALE (ESS)

Name: ....

Today's date: ....   Sex: Male/Female

Age: ....

Height: ....   Weight: ....

Each item below describes a routine daytime situation.

Use the scale below to rate the likelihood that you would doze off or fall asleep (in contrast to just feeling tired) during that activity.

If you haven't done some of these things recently, consider how you think they would affect you.

Use the following scale to choose the most appropriate number for each situation:

0	1	2	3
Would never doze	Slight chance of dozing	Moderate chance of dozing	High chance of dozing

Watching TV	Chance of dozing ....
Sitting inactive in a public place, for example a theatre or meeting	Chance of dozing ....
In a car, while stopped in traffic	Chance of dozing ....
Sitting and reading	Chance of dozing ....
Sitting and talking to someone	Chance of dozing ....
As a passenger in a car without a break for an hour	Chance of dozing ....
Lying down to rest in the afternoon	Chance of dozing ....
Sitting quietly after lunch when you've had no alcohol	Chance of dozing ....

3.23 The Epworth Sleepiness Scale. A useful screening tool for obstructive sleep apnoea in conjunction with symptoms of snoring and apnoeas during sleep. A score of ≥11 supports the diagnosis (with permission[21]).

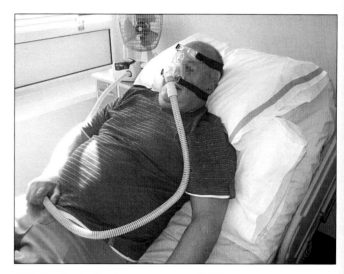

3.24 A patient with sleep apnoea on CPAP therapy.

Thrombo-embolic disease

Obesity more than doubles the risk of pulmonary embolism and deep venous thrombosis. This may be in part due to the more sedentary lifestyle that many obese subjects follow, but also due to venous stasis that arises from increased intra-abdominal pressure and the hypercoagulable state associated with obesity (increased levels of factor VIII and von Willebrand factor are seen in obese subjects).

Renal disease

Obesity is closely linked to chronic kidney disease directly and indirectly (**3.26**). In addition to its indirect effects on the renovascular system through its association with vascular risk factors such as hypertension and dyslipidaemia, obesity has been shown to directly cause several functional alterations in renal physiology that may eventually lead to renal glomerulosclerosis.[21]

In a large epidemiological study, overweight (BMI ≥25 kg/m^2) at age 20 was associated with a significant threefold excess risk for chronic renal failure, relative to BMI <25 kg/m^2 (*Table 3.9*).[22] Obesity (BMI ≥30 kg/m^2) among men and morbid obesity (BMI ≥35 kg/m^2) among women at any time during their lifetime was linked to three- to fourfold increases in risk. The strongest association was with diabetic nephropathy, but two- to threefold risk elevations were observed for all major subtypes of chronic renal failure.

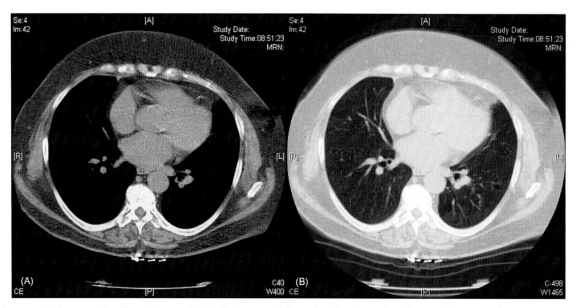

3.25 Chest computed tomography of an obese patient with hypoventilation, chronic obstructive airways disease, and pulmonary hypertension.

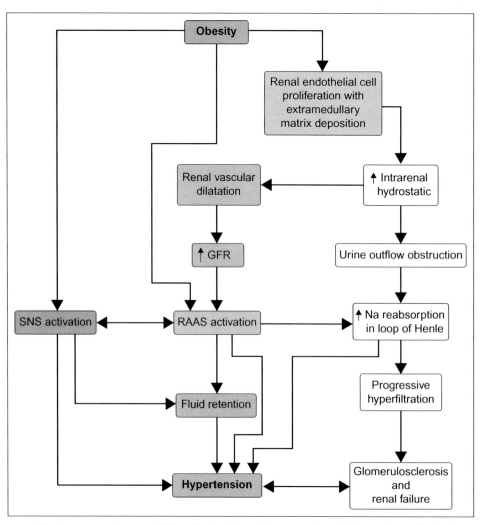

3.26 Mechanisms responsible for progressive renal failure in obesity and hypertension (with permission[23]). GFR, glomerular filtration rate; Na, sodium; RAAS, renin–angiotensin–aldosterone system; SNS, sympathetic nervous system.

Table 3.9 Risk of CRF with obesity[22]

Body mass index range	Odds ratio for CRF	
	Men	Women
<25	1.0	1.0
25–29.9	1.4	1.2
30–34.9	2.7	1.4
>35	4.4	3.1

CRF, chronic renal failure.

Fertility and pregnancy

The effects of obesity on fertility and obesity are summarized below.

Male fertility
- Reduced total and free testosterone blood concentration.
- Reduced androstenedione and dihydrotestosterone levels.
- Reduced sex hormone-binding globulin (SHBG) concentration.
- Impaired secretion of the hypothalamic gonadotrophin-releasing hormone.
- Increased oestrogen production in response to body weight.
- Increased leptin concentration.
- Reduced spermatogenesis and subfertility.
- Erectile dysfunction (independent of the effects of diabetes).

Female fertility
- Impaired pubertal development related to childhood and adolescent obesity.
- Earlier menarche.
- Reduced ovulation.
- Increased incidence of menstrual irregularities.
- Subfertility and reduced conception rates.
- Hyperandrogenism.
- Reduced luteinizing hormone (LH) concentrations.
- Polycystic ovarian syndrome associated with reduced fertility, menstrual irregularities, hyperinsulinaemia, and hyperandrogenism.

Pregnancy and assisted conception
- Increased risk of miscarriages.

- Effects on the function of the corpus luteum and that of trophoblast function, early embryo development and endometrial receptivity.
- Unfavourable effect on follicle growth, embryo development, and implantation.
- Poor outcomes following ovulation induction and assisted reproductive therapy.
- Higher risk of obstetric causes of maternal death and anaesthesia-related deaths.
- Higher rates of complications in pregnancy, mainly in the third trimester, such as hypertension, pre-eclampsia, gestational diabetes, thrombo-embolism, anaemia, urinary tract infection, preterm labour, and delivery.
- Higher sudden and unexplained intrauterine death, operative vaginal deliveries, caesarean section delivery, and anaesthetic and surgical complications.
- Increased postpartum haemorrhage, postoperative wound infection and dehiscence, and endomyometritis in the puerperium.
- Fetal macrosomia and malformations such as defects of the central nervous system (neural tube defects), great vessels, ventral wall, and intestine.
- Children of obese mothers run a higher risk of intrauterine fetal death, head trauma, shoulder dystocia, brachial plexus lesions, fractures of the clavicle, meconium aspiration, fetal distress, and increased risk of death in the first year.
- Reduced breast-feeding.
- Fetal adiposity and increased risk of obesity in the child.

Gastrointestinal diseases

- Fatty liver, steatohepatitis.
- Gastro-oesophageal reflux disease.
- Gallstones, cholecystitis.
- Altered bowel habits.

Cancer and obesity

There is growing evidence from epidemiological and observational studies that obesity is associated with increased risk of cancer and cancer-related mortality (**3.27**, *Table 3.10*). Several studies have shown strong associations between BMI and numerous cancers but the exact mechanisms underlying this are still unclear. It also remains to be seen if subsequent weight loss and lifestyle change have any impact on cancer incidence or severity.

Million Women study[24] (**3.27**) was a prospective cohort study to examine the relationship between body mass index and cancer incidence and mortality. Between 1996 and 2001, 1.2 million UK women aged between 50 and 64 were recruited into the study and were followed up, on average, for 5.4 years for cancer incidence and 7.0 years for cancer mortality. Increasing body mass index was associated with an increased incidence of endometrial cancer (trend in relative risk per 10 units was 2.89), adenocarcinoma of the oesophagus (2.38), kidney cancer (1.53), leukaemia (1.50), multiple myeloma (1.31), pancreatic cancer (1.24), non-Hodgkin lymphoma (1.17), ovarian cancer (1.14), all cancers combined (1.12), breast cancer in postmenopausal women (1.40) and colorectal cancer in premenopausal women (1.61). In general, the relationship between body mass index and cancer-related mortality was similar to that for incidence of cancer. 5% of all cancers in postmenopausal women in the UK (about 6000 annually) are attributable to being overweight or obese. Body mass index is a significant modifiable risk factor for endometrial cancer and adenocarcinoma of the oesophagus and about half of all cases in postmenopausal women are attributable to overweight or obesity.

Musculoskeletal

People who are overweight or obese are at an increased risk of musculoskeletal disorders such as chronic joint pain and osteoarthritis (OA) leading to problems with posture, activities of daily living, and mobility. Commonly affected areas are the weight-bearing joints such as knees, hips, ankles, feet, and lower back (**3.28, 3.29**), but there is also increased incidence of problems in shoulders, hands, upper back, and neck. Being overweight increases the load placed on the weight-bearing joints such as the knee, which increases the stress and could possibly hasten the breakdown of cartilage. Data from the first National Health and Nutrition Examination Survey (NHANES I) indicated that obese women had nearly four times the risk of knee OA as compared with non-obese women; for obese men, the risk was nearly five times greater. It is estimated that persons in the highest quintile of body weight have up to 10 times the risk of knee OA than those in the lowest quintile. Several studies have shown that even small amounts of weight loss reduce the risk of developing knee OA. Some preliminary studies suggest weight loss decreases pain substantially in those with knee OA.

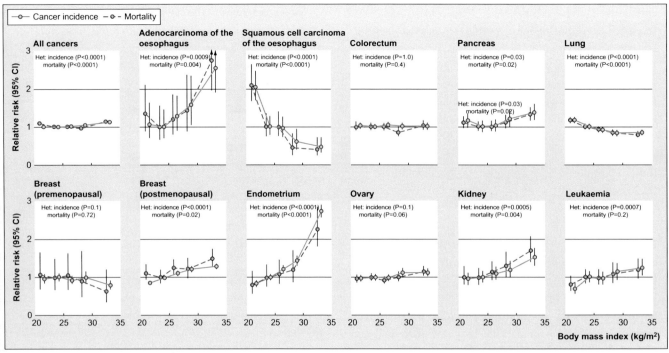

3.27 Million Women Study. Relative risk of cancer incidence and mortality for individual cancer sites or types according to BMI (22.5–24.9 = reference group). Adjusted for age, geographical region, socio-economic status, age at first birth, parity, smoking status, alcohol intake, physical activity, and, where appropriate, time since menopause and use of hormone replacement therapy (with permission[24]).
* = restricted to never users of hormone replacement therapy; Het = test for heterogeneity across categories of BMI on df = 4.

Table 3.10 Relative risks associated with overweight and obesity, and the percentage of cases attributable to overweight and obesity in the USA and European Union (EU)[25]

Type of cancer	Relative risk with BMI of 25–30 kg/m²	Relative risk with BMI of ≥30 kg/m²	PAF (%) for US population†	PAF (%) for EU population‡
Colorectal (men)	1.5	2.0	35.4	27.5
Colorectal (women)	1.2	1.5	20.8	14.2
Female breast (postmenopausal)	1.3	1.5	22.6	16.7
Endometrial	2.0	3.5	56.8	45.2
Kidney (renal cell)	1.5	2.5	42.5	31.1
Oesophageal (adenocarcinoma)	2.0	3.0	52.4	42.7
Pancreatic	1.3	1.7	26.9	19.3
Liver	ND	1.5–4.0	ND	ND
Gallbladder	1.5	2.0	35.5	37.1
Gastric cardia (adenocarcinoma)	1.5	2.0	35.5	27.1

*Relative risk estimates are summarized from the literature cited in reference 25. †Data on prevalence of overweight and obesity are from the National Health and Nutrition Examination Survey (1999–2000) for men and women from the USA aged from 50 to 69 years. ‡Data on prevalence of overweight and obesity are from a range of sources for adult men and women residing in 15 European countries in the 1980s and 1990s.
BMI, body mass index; ND, not determined; PAF, population attributable fraction.

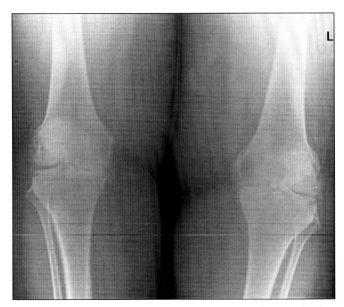

3.28 X-ray of knees showing osteoarthritis secondary to obesity.

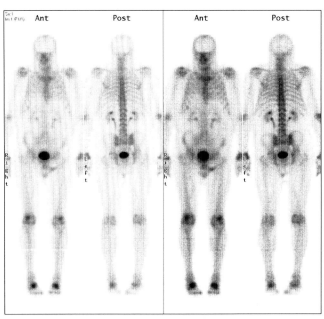

3.29 Isotope bone scan of obese subject with increased uptake in weight-bearing joints showing generalized degenerative arthritis.

Neurological and psychosocial

Cerebrovascular disease

Obesity increases the risk of cerebrovascular disease independently as well through its association with hypertension, dyslipidaemia, insulin resistance, and diabetes. In a recent study, the prevalence of stroke was found to be significantly higher in middle-aged women who participated in the National Health and Nutrition Examination Survey (NHANES) IV study when compared with the NHANES III population. The only difference between the two groups was higher BMI and waist circumference; in fact, other risk factors such as dyslipidaemia and blood pressure were better controlled in the NHANES IV group than the NHANES III group.

Other neurological conditions associated with obesity

- Dementia.
- Autonomic nervous system dysfunction.
- Frequency and severity of migraines.
- Parkinson's disease.
- Benign intracranial hypertension.
- Carpal tunnel syndrome.

Psychosocial effects (3.30)

- Depressive illness and anxiety.
- Low self-esteem.
- Daytime sleepiness.
- Fatigue.
- Body dysmorphic disorder.
- Social stigmatization.

Miscellaneous

Obesity increases the risk of developing varicose veins and venous ulcers. Obesity is associated with increased intra-abdominal pressure and poor blood flow in leg veins leading to enlargement of the veins and valve incompetence. Deep venous thrombosis also can damage the valves permanently. This, along with chronic lymphoedema, increases the risk of recurrent cellulitis, leg ulcers, and venous eczema (**3.31–3.33**).

Examination of obese people can often show markers of insulin resistance such as acanthosis nigricans, a brown–black, poorly defined, velvety hyperpigmentation of the skin,

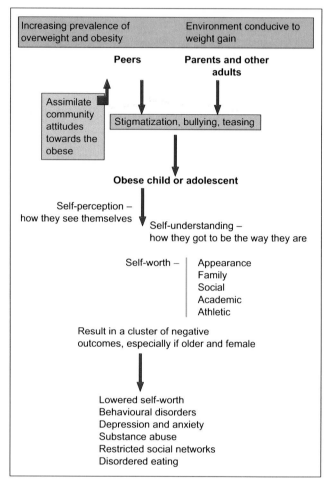

3.30 The psychosocial world of the obese child and adolescent (with permission[26]).

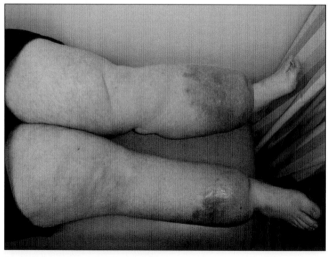

3.31 Lymphoedema and cellulitis.

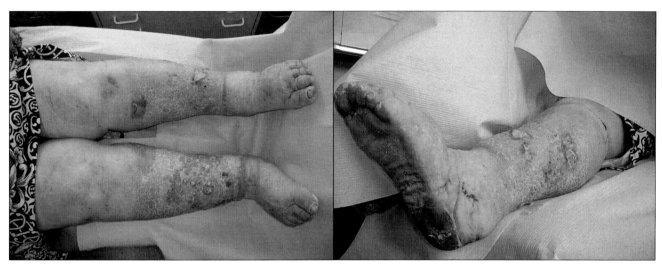

3.32 Venous oedema, pressure ulcers, and cellulitis.

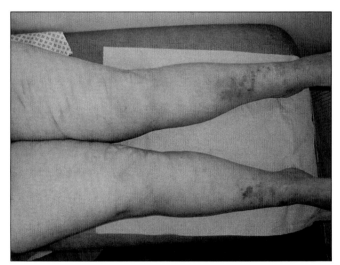

3.33 Varicose veins.

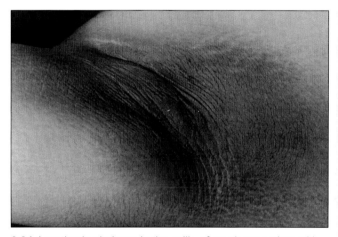

3.34 Acanthosis nigricans in the axilla of an obese patient with severe insulin resistance.

usually present in the posterior and lateral folds of the neck, the axilla, groin, umbilicus, and other areas (**3.34**), which is also associated with type 2 diabetes and polycystic ovarian syndrome. Obese men can also have pseudo-gynaecomastia (**3.35**), which is due to excess fat deposition in the chest. True gynaecomastia, which is usually related to endocrine disorders, is due to increased breast glandular tissue but pseudo-gynaecomastia is an increase in adipose tissue in the chest without increased glandular tissue.

Obese people often have mobility problems secondary to musculoskeletal disorders and peripheral vascular disease as discussed before. They also are prone to chronic leg oedema and its associated complications. The chronic oedema could

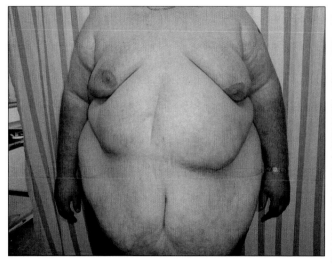

3.35 Pseudo-gynaecomastia in morbid obesity.

be due to impaired lymphatic and/or venous circulation. This makes them prone to eczema, stasis ulcers, recurrent cellulitis, and thrombo-embolism.

Increased weight is a well-recognized risk factor for developing inguinal and abdominal hernia (**3.36**, **3.37**). Obese people are also prone to developing incisional hernias, which could be difficult to repair. Surgeons often avoid surgery to correct these due to the high recurrence rates and advise people to lose weight to improve chances of success.

Associations of obesity with cataracts, glaucoma, age-related maculopathy, and retinopathy have been reported with varying degrees of certainty.

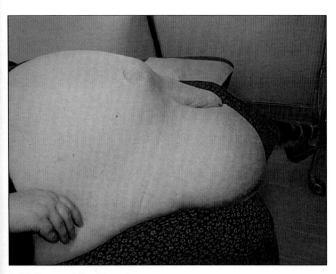

3.36 Paraumbilical hernia.

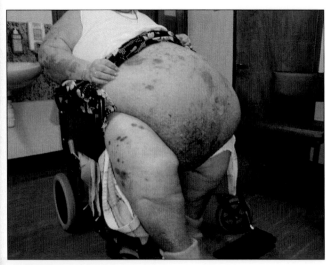

3.37 Massive abdominal hernia.

References

1. Miranda PJ, DeFronzo RA, Califf RM, Guyton JR. Metabolic syndrome: definition, pathophysiology, and mechanisms. *Am Heart J* 2005; **149**: 33–45.

2. Definition, Diagnosis and Classification of Diabetes Mellitus and its Complications. Report of a WHO Consultation. WHO 1999.

3. Executive Summary of The Third Report of The National Cholesterol Education Program (NCEP) Expert Panel on Detection, Evaluation, And Treatment of High Blood Cholesterol In Adults (Adult Treatment Panel III). *JAMA* 2001; **285**: 2486–97.

4. The IDF Consensus Worldwide Definition of the Metabolic Syndrome. International Diabetes Federation, 2006.

5. Grundy SM, Cleeman JI, Daniels SR, *et al.* Diagnosis and management of the metabolic syndrome: an American Heart Association/National Heart, Lung, and Blood Institute Scientific Statement. *Circulation* 2005; **112**: 2735–52.

6. Reaven G. Syndrome X: 10 years after. *Drugs* 1999; **58**(Suppl 1): 19–20.

7. Ramlo-Halsted BA, Edelman SV. The natural history of type 2 diabetes. Implications for clinical practice. *Prim Care* 1999; **26**: 771–89.

8. Paradisi G, Smith L, Burtner C, *et al.* Dual energy X–ray absorptiometry assessment of fat mass distribution and its association with the insulin resistance syndrome. *Diabetes Care* 1999; **22**: 1310–17.

9. Chan JM, Rimm EB, Colditz GA, Stampfer MJ, Willett WC. Obesity, fat distribution, and weight gain as risk factors for clinical diabetes in men. *Diabetes Care* 1994; **17**: 961–9.

10. Colditz GA, Willett WC, Stampfer MJ, *et al.* Weight as a risk factor for clinical diabetes in women. *Am J Epidemiol* 1990; **132**: 501–13.

11. Alexander CM, Landsman PB, Teutsch SM, Haffner SM. NCEP-defined metabolic syndrome, diabetes, and prevalence of coronary heart disease among NHANES III participants age 50 years and older. *Diabetes* 2003; **52**: 1210–14.

12. Bays HE, Bazata DD, Clark NG, *et al.* Prevalence of self-reported diagnosis of diabetes mellitus and associated risk factors in a national survey in the US population: SHIELD (Study to Help Improve Early evaluation and management of risk factors Leading to Diabetes). *BMC Public Health* 2007; **7**: 277.

13. Despres JP, Lemieux I. Abdominal obesity and metabolic syndrome. *Nature* 2006; **444**: 881–7.
14. Pouliot MC, Despres JP, Nadeau A, *et al.* Visceral obesity in men. Associations with glucose tolerance, plasma insulin, and lipoprotein levels. *Diabetes* 1992; **41**: 826–34.
15. Stevens J, Cai J, Evenson KR, Thomas R. Fitness and fatness as predictors of mortality from all causes and from cardiovascular disease in men and women in the lipid research clinics study. *Am J Epidemiol* 2002; **156**: 832–41.
16. Rexrode KM, Carey VJ, Hennekens CH, *et al.* Abdominal adiposity and coronary heart disease in women. *JAMA* 1998; **280**: 1843–8.
17. Aneja A, El-Atat F, McFarlane SI, Sowers JR. Hypertension and obesity. *Recent Prog Horm Res* 2004; **59**: 169–205.
18. Yusuf S, Hawken S, Ounpuu S, *et al.* Effect of potentially modifiable risk factors associated with myocardial infarction in 52 countries (the INTERHEART study): case-control study. *Lancet* 2004; **364**: 937–52.
19. Van Gaal LF, Mertens IL, De Block CE. Mechanisms linking obesity with cardiovascular disease. *Nature* 2006; **444**: 875–80.
20. Kenchaiah S, Evans JC, Levy D, *et al.* Obesity and the risk of heart failure. *N Engl J Med* 2002; **347**: 305–13.
21. Johns MW. A new method for measuring daytime sleepiness: the Epworth sleepiness scale. *Sleep* 1991; **14**: 540–45.
22. Rocchini AP, Key J, Bondie D, *et al.* The effect of weight loss on the sensitivity of blood pressure to sodium in obese adolescents. *N Engl J Med* 1989; **321**: 580–5.
23. Ejerblad E, Fored CM, Lindblad P, *et al.* Obesity and risk for chronic renal failure. *J Am Soc Nephrol* 2006; **17**: 1695–702.
24. Reeves GK, Pirie K, Beral V, *et al.* Cancer incidence and mortality in relation to body mass index in the Million Women Study: cohort study. *BMJ* 2007; **335**: 1134.
25. Calle EE, Kaaks R. Overweight, obesity and cancer: epidemiological evidence and proposed mechanisms. *Nat Rev Cancer* 2004; 4: 579–91.
26. Peter Kopelman ICWD. *Clinical Obesity in Adults and Children*, 2nd edn. Blackwell Publishing. 2005.

Management of obesity

Assessment of the obese patient

Healthcare professionals are beginning to realize that obesity is a major preventable health risk. It is strongly associated, directly and indirectly, with a wide variety of health problems and is recognized as a significant risk factor for serious morbidity and mortality (*see* Chapter 3). The aetiology of obesity is complex and multifactorial and, therefore, a detailed and thorough assessment of an obese patient is an essential first step in successful management. In addition to careful assessment of the lifestyle of an individual, the aim is to rule out genetic and neuroendocrine causes of obesity, to assess the presence and extent of comorbidities, to arrange further medical and laboratory investigations, and to determine the individual's risk of complications of obesity such as cardiovascular disease, diabetes, and sleep apnoea. *Table 4.1* summarizes essential steps in the assessment of an obese individual. This assessment is crucial in deciding an appropriate management plan and recognizing the possible complications that may arise from treatment. Often, the most difficult step is evaluating the individual's motivation and readiness for weight loss and the potential 'barriers' to change. It is essential to remember that the focus of the assessment and management plan has to be tailored to each individual's problems and needs.

Measures of body fatness and fat distribution (see Chapter 1)
- Height.
- Weight.
- Body mass index (BMI).
- Waist circumference (if BMI <35 kg/m^2; *see* Chapter 1).
- Bioelectrical impedance analysis (if available).

Physical examination
- Blood pressure (BP; using an appropriately sized cuff).
- Detailed examination of all systems with a high level of suspicion of obesity-related comorbidities and complications.
- Assessment of mobility and dependence in activities of daily living.

Laboratory assessment
Not all tests are recommended routinely but they should be considered if the patient's history or examination is suggestive.

- Random/fasting blood sugar.
- Fasting lipid profile.
- Renal profile (may require urine dipstick, protein estimation, and microscopy).
- Liver profile (ultrasound scan of liver if indicated).
- Serum thyroid-stimulating hormone if hypothyroidism suspected.
- Overnight dexamethasone suppression test (ODST) to rule out Cushing's syndrome.
- Sex hormone profile if subfertility, menstrual irregularities, or polycystic ovary syndrome.
- Sleep studies (polysomnography and/or overnight oximetry).
- Arrange genetic screening (*see* Chapter 2) if high suspicion or young age of onset of obesity.

Assessment of risk
All the above information will determine the individual's overall risk status and the level of need for clinical intervention. The management plan must be discussed in detail with the patient to facilitate understanding and cooperation. The success of management of obesity is heavily dependent on the patient's motivation and willingness to change. Agreeing reasonable weight loss goals and a strategy for weight maintenance is also essential (*Table 4.2*).

Table 4.1 Assessment of an obese individual

History
- Reasons for wanting to lose weight
- Understanding of causes and risks of obesity
- Motivation and readiness to change
- Perceptions, beliefs, and potential barriers to change
- Expectations and targets

Factors predisposing to obesity
- Family history of obesity and related comorbidities
- History suggestive of endocrine disorders (e.g. hypothyroidism, Cushing's syndrome, polycystic ovarian syndrome, acromegaly) and neuroendocrine causes such as central nervous system injury
- Dietary pattern (e.g. meal times and frequency, dependence on high calorie foods, portion sizes, comfort eating, night eating, binges, and eating disorders)
- Physical activity and daily routine
- Assessment of mental status (mood), psychosocial influences, well-being, and quality of life
- Lifestyle changes concurrent with onset of weight gain (e.g. marriage, divorce, employment, childbirth)

Medical diseases
- History of current medical conditions and risk factors
- History of possible comorbidities and complications of obesity (e.g. diabetes, cardiovascular disease, sleep apnoea)
- Smoking history, alcohol and recreational substance use
- Reproductive history (menstrual irregularities, fertility, polycystic ovary syndrome)

Drug treatment
- Medication(s) contributing to weight gain (e.g. steroids, beta-blockers, antidepressants, antipsychotics, anticonvulsants, diabetes treatment, hormone therapy)
- Previous use of slimming pills and aids (prescribed, over-the-counter, and unlicensed products)

Past weight loss attempts and outcomes
- Onset of weight gain and progression
- Details of previous attempts (including failed attempts)
- Successes and relapses
- Problems with weight maintenance
- Impact on confidence and motivation

Factors warranting precaution (needing specialized care)
- Possible genetic disorders or secondary causes (endocrine, gastrointestinal, and neurological)
- History of eating disorders or significant disordered eating habits
- History of substance abuse
- Uncontrolled major psychiatric illnesses and behavioural problems
- Pregnancy and lactation
- Presence of serious illnesses where energy restriction is not recommended

Table 4.2 Aims and goals of obesity treatment

- 5–10% weight loss is a reasonable medium-term goal for most patients
- Improve appearance and self-esteem
- Reduce risk to health and complications
- Improve existing comorbidities (e.g. diabetes control, heart disease, sleep apnoea)
- Improve activity, mobility, and independence in activities of daily living
- Improve well-being, quality of life, and productivity
- Individual goals (e.g. occupational, special occasions, eligibility for surgery)

Dietary interventions

The education of an obese patient about diet and eating habits is an essential component of any weight loss treatment. Commercial diets and dietary intervention-based weight loss programmes have gained a lot of popularity and acceptance in recent years. However, the general perceptions about dietary intervention for weight loss are often skewed from the basic principles of dietary management. These dietary interventions are usually effective in the short term but their lack of effectiveness in the long term is well documented. The diet cycle (**4.1**) is a common problem faced by obese subjects and ways to break the 'yo-yo' dieting culture should be part of the management plan. *Table 4.3* summarizes the different approaches in dietary management.

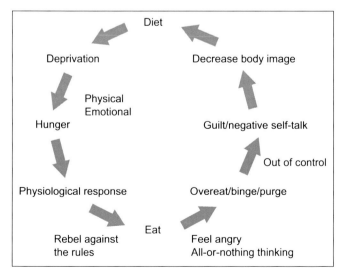

4.1 'The Diet Cycle' (with permission[1]).

Calorie restriction and reduced portion sizes are important to achieve weight loss but dietary advice should also include the importance of a well balanced diet. The 'eatwell plate' recommended by the Food Standards Agency (UK) highlights the importance of a balanced diet and the essential components of a healthy one (**4.2**).

An appropriate dietary management plan is essential for the success of any weight loss intervention such as the use of anti-obesity drugs or bariatric surgery; dietary intervention is very important in long-term weight loss maintenance. It is also worth remembering that the success of dietary management depends on careful assessment of every subject, particularly the recognition of behavioural problems (e.g. eating disorders) and readiness to change (*Table 4.4*).

Physical exercise

Exercise is an essential adjunct to the successful management of obesity. 'Energy expenditure' is as important as 'energy restriction' in achieving 'energy balance'. There are also weight-loss-independent beneficial health effects of exercise in obesity (*Table 4.5*). Several comorbidities related to obesity are also improved, and obesity-induced complications can be avoided by modest exercise. The role of physical exercise in obesity prevention and long-term weight loss maintenance cannot be overemphasized. Obese subjects should be educated on the importance of improving cardiovascular 'fitness' rather than just focusing on measures of 'fatness' such as body weight and dress size.

The only way to accurately measure total daily energy expenditure is by the doubly labelled water technique. It is possible to determine resting metabolic rate (e.g. using a calorimeter) and thermic effect of food (15% of total). By subtracting these from total energy expenditure, an estimate of energy expenditure by physical activity can be made (*see* Chapter 2—the 'energy pyramid'). It is not practical to use this technique in large observational studies; questionnaires that estimate physical activity (in units such as METs, or metabolic equivalents) are used instead. Lower levels of physical activity are strongly related to weight gain in several large studies (e.g. NHANES I, Multiple Risk Factor Intervention Trial (MRFIT)). The importance of physical activity in the prevention of weight gain is discussed in Chapter 5.

The amount and type of exercise required depends on the goals of the programme being followed (*Table 4.6*). Aerobic exercises are usually recommended, but the intensity of exercise will depend on several factors, including

Table 4.3 Approaches to dietary management of obesity

- *Modest calorie deficit diet.* A 500–1000 kcal deficit from usual daily intake should lead to approximately 0.5–1 kg weight loss per week. This is often combined with drug treatment and behavioural therapy. This plan can improve compliance by offering flexibility and is less rigid than other diets.

- *Fixed energy diet.* A strict dietary plan is provided to limit the energy intake to 1200 kcal for women and 1800 kcal/ day for men by controlling portion sizes and limiting menu choice and composition.

- *Ad libitum diet (self-limiting).* Patients are encouraged to self-limit one or all dietary constituents to maintain carbohydrate intake to 55% of diet, fat 30%, and 15% as protein irrespective of their calorie intake. These are possibly better at weight maintenance than most restrictive diets.

- *Low calorie diets.* Calorie intake is restricted to 800–1200 kcal/day. They are not recommended without medical supervision and patients may need supplementation of essential nutrients. Long-term compliance is often the limiting factor.

- *VLCD.* Calorie intake is restricted to 400–800 kcal/day for a fixed period only. They include daily supplementation of minerals, vitamins, electrolytes, and fatty acids. They require very close monitoring due to risk of serious complications. Compliance is a major drawback like any other restrictive diet and long-term follow-up studies have failed to show any additional benefit over other diets (**4.3**). Routine use is not recommended but in special situations (e.g. pre-surgery) they may be useful in achieving targets. They are available commercially but can be quite expensive (e.g. Lipotrim, Lighter Life).

- *Low fat diets.* They cause weight loss proportional to pretreatment weight and to long-term reduction in fat content. They also have a beneficial effect on cardiovascular risk factors. Strict adherence to a low fat diet is advised to minimize the gastrointestinal side effects with the use of intestinal lipase inhibitors such as orlistat.

- *High protein diets.* More than 20% of total energy consumed comes from protein; very high protein diet provides more than 30% of energy intake. Low carbohydrate diet (less than 40% of energy comes from carbohydrates) is often combined. They induce ketogenesis and produce weight loss due to fluid depletion and suppression of appetite. Their effect on lipid profile is debated.

- *Low GI diet.* The GI is determined by measuring the area under the blood glucose curve (effect on postprandial glucose levels) in comparison with reference food with equal carbohydrate content. The GI of a food will depend on the rate of digestion (low <50 and high >70). Although the effectiveness of a low GI diet in causing significant weight loss has not yet been determined, they appear to have beneficial effects on lipid profile and insulin sensitivity.

- *Meal replacements.* Usually two of three meals a day (breakfast and lunch) are replaced by functional foods in the form of drinks, soups, or cereal bars. Most plans also allow the use of one or two snacks in between. These meal replacements provide a lower calorie intake than conventional meals (but more calories than a VLCD diet) and a more complete profile of micronutrients. It is better than skipping meals and compliance is better as it allows one conventional meal of about 600 kcal/day. There is some evidence from studies in the USA and Germany about their effectiveness and safety (**4.4**). There are several companies that market these products (e.g. Slimfast) but the cost of treatment and compliance issues must be taken into consideration before they are recommended.

- *Commercial slimming clubs, self-help groups, and special diet programmes.* These are gaining in popularity and although most commercial groups (e.g. 'Weight Watchers' and 'Slimming World') provide advice consistent with standard recommendations such as those from Food Standards Agency, National Institute for Health and Clinical Excellence, etc., there is very limited controlled evidence about the effectiveness, safety, and long-term achievements of some programmes. Obese subjects should be encouraged to ensure that the weight-loss programme they choose is safe and suitable to their needs. Certain 'health foods' and 'crash dieting programmes' can be harmful and the need for tighter regulation and monitoring has been raised in recent years.

GI, glycaemic index; VLCD, Very low calorie diets.

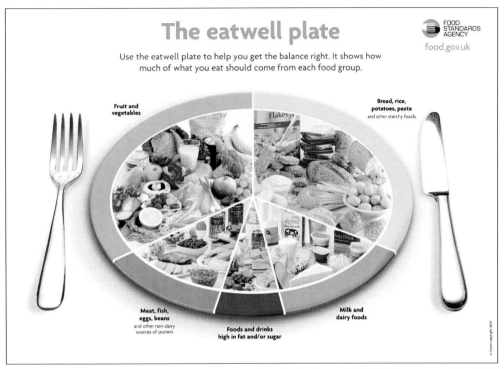

4.2 The 'eatwell plate' recommended by the Food Standards Agency (UK) (© Crown copyright 2007).

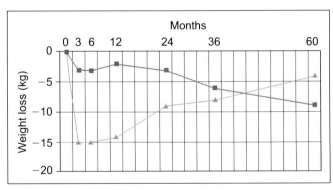

4.3 Long-term weight changes following conventional diets and very low calorie diets (mean weight loss over 5 years after intensive self-selected diet treatments: ▲, 13 diabetic subjects after very low calorie diet; ■, 12 diabetic subjects after intensive conventional diet) (with permission[3]).

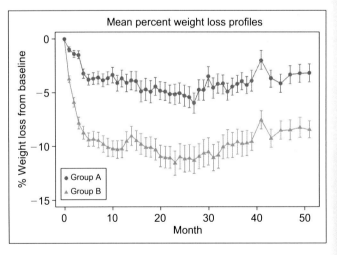

4.4 Weight loss achieved with meal replacement therapy in comparison with conventional diet and long-term maintenance (with permission[2]). Mean (±SEM) percentage change from initial body weight in patients during 51 months of treatment with an energy-restricted diet (1200–1500 kcal/day). Data were analysed on an available case basis. Patients received either a conventional energy-restricted diet (control Group A, ●) or a diet with two meal and snack replacements (Group B, ▲) for 3 months. During the remaining 4 years, all patients received one meal and snack replacement daily.

Table 4.4 Common problems in dietary management

- Compliance
- Under reporting of intake
- Underdiagnosis of binges and eating disorders
- Lack of confidence due to previous failures and common negative perceptions
- Mixed messages
- Cost
- Lack of flexibility
- Problems with weight maintenance after initial weight loss and lack of long-term evidence

Table 4.5 Health benefits of exercise

- Prevention of weight gain
- Reduce or maintain body weight or body fat (particularly reduce abdominal fat)
- Improved cardiovascular and cardiorespiratory fitness
- Building and maintaining healthy bone density, muscle strength, and joint mobility
- Promoting physiological well-being
- Reduce risk of premature death and all-cause mortality risk
- Reduce the risk of developing and/or dying from ischaemic heart disease and stroke
- Reduce high blood pressure or the risk of developing high blood pressure
- Improve lipid profile ($\downarrow$ triglycerides, $\uparrow$ high-density lipoprotein)
- Improve haemostatic factors associated with thrombosis
- Reduce the risk of developing diabetes and improve insulin resistance
- Reduce depression and anxiety and improve psychological well-being
- Enhanced work, recreation, and sport performance
- Improved strength, balance, and functional ability in older adults

Table 4.6 Types of exercise

Flexibility exercises	e.g. stretching, which improve the range of motion of muscles and joints
Aerobic exercises	e.g. cycling, walking, running, hiking, which focus on increasing respiratory and cardiovascular endurance
Anaerobic exercises	e.g. sprinting, weight training, and functional training to increase short-term muscle strength and function

Table 4.7 Intensity of exercise

Light exercise	Activity that allows one to talk at the same time (e.g. walking, light housework, gardening)
Moderate exercise	Makes one feel slightly out of breath and slightly worn out, but not to the extent where it is unbearable (e.g. brisk walking, walking up a hill)
Vigorous exercise	Makes one breathe rapidly; feels like one is just at the point where they are pushing their body's boundaries, without doing any harm (e.g. jogging, cycling, swimming, and weight training)

interventions, drugs, and behavioural therapy (**4.5**). There are numerous additional benefits such as improved fitness (cardiac, respiratory, orthopaedic, and psychological), favourable changes in body composition, reduced cardiovascular risk, and improvements in comorbidities and quality of life (QOL) (**4.6**). Regular physical activity is an important factor in the maintenance of weight loss after any intervention.

Recommendations: points to remember

- Endurance exercise (aerobic) training induces modest weight and fat loss, which is more pronounced in overweight than in lean individuals.
- When combined with diet control, people who exercise regularly are shown to lose more weight and are more likely to maintain weight loss.

the functional ability of the individual and the presence of limiting comorbidities (*Table 4.7*).

There are several studies that have evaluated the effect of exercise in inducing weight loss. Although the weight loss attributed to exercise alone is very small, there are plenty of data to support the use of exercise in addition to dietary

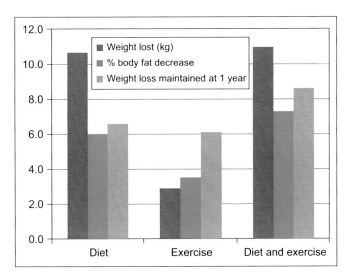

4.5 Changes in body weight, body fat percentage, and weight maintenance in obese adults following diet, exercise, or combined therapy (with permission[4]).

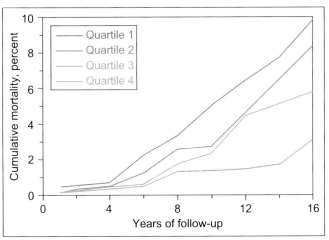

4.6 Mortality from cardiovascular disease according to fitness quartile: cumulative age-adjusted mortality from cardiovascular causes (over 16 years follow-up) was inversely proportional to fitness quartile in healthy, middle-aged Norwegian men (with permission[5]).

- Resistance (anaerobic) training has very little effect on weight, but increases fat-free mass and functional capacity.
- Dynamic exercise with large muscle groups is recommended; moderate intensity physical activity for 30 minutes on a daily basis or 45–60 minutes three times a week is recommended for weight management. However, 45–60 minutes of moderate intensity exercise per day is needed to prevent the transition from overweight to obesity and 60–90 minutes/day to prevent weight regain after successful weight loss.

- Compliance problems with exercise programmes should be addressed at regular intervals.
- Current functional capacity and the presence of comorbidities and complications should be taken into consideration when recommending exercise routines.
- A gradual increase in the intensity and duration of exercise should be recommended to avoid exercise-related injuries in obese subjects.
- Individuals with morbid obesity or obesity with serious comorbidities may need careful assessment and monitoring by physiotherapists or specialist fitness therapists.

Behavioural therapy and eating disorders

Behavioural therapy for weight management focuses on the modification of people's eating habits and their level of physical activity. Careful assessment of a particular individual's causes of weight gain or inability to lose weight or maintain weight loss should identify the need for behavioural treatment. Failure of weight management with lifestyle modifications or drugs should alert the physician to investigate the presence of an eating disorder or compliance problems. Subjects with clear-cut eating disorders are best managed in specialized centres, but successful weight management plans should involve at least some degree of behavioural modification.

Eating disorders related to overweight and obesity

1. Bulimia nervosa (atypical type sometimes associated with overweight). (Please refer to DSM-IV and ICD-10 definitions for diagnostic criteria.)
   - Recurrent episodes of overeating (at least twice a week for 3 months).
   - Persistent preoccupation with eating (strong desire or sense of compulsion to eat).
   - Inappropriate compensatory habits: self-induced vomiting; misuse of laxatives, diuretics, enemas, or other drugs; periods of starvation; and excessive exercise.
   - Self-perception of being fat and a dread of fatness.
2. Binge eating disorder
   - Recurrent episodes of binge eating (large amounts in a discrete period of time with a lack of control over eating during the episode).

- Associated with at least three of the following:
  - eating more rapidly than normal.
  - eating until feeling uncomfortably full.
  - eating large amounts even when not hungry.
  - eating alone because of embarrassment.
  - feeling disgusted, depressed, or very guilty after overeating.
- Marked distress regarding binge eating is present.
- Occurs, on average, at least 2 days a week for 6 months.
- Not associated with the regular use of inappropriate compensatory behaviour.
3. Night-eating syndrome
4. Anxiety, depression-related eating disorders
5. Addictive disorders affecting eating habits
6. Personality and eating disorders

Components of behavioural therapy for obesity (4.7)[6]

- Self-monitoring is the most important component of behavioural therapy for obesity and involves keeping daily records of food intake and physical activity, as well as checking weight regularly. Self-monitoring records can provide information needed to identify links in the behaviour chain that can be targeted for intervention. In addition, record keeping enhances compliance with dietary and physical activity interventions.
- Problem solving is a systematic method of analysing problems and identifying possible solutions.

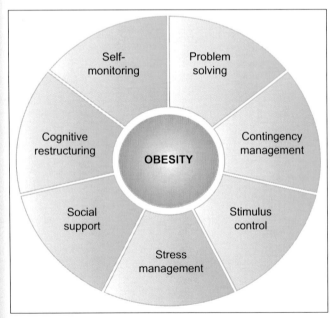

4.7 Cognitive behaviour therapy (CBT) components (with permission[6]).

- Contingency management involves developing methods to help recovery from episodes of overeating or weight regain.
- Stimulus control is the process of avoiding triggers that prompt eating.
- Stress management is used to decrease the negative impact of stress on positive behaviour patterns.
- Social support from family members and friends is important for modifying lifestyle and behaviour.
- Cognitive restructuring teaches patients to think in a positive way and correct thoughts that undermine weight management efforts. Cognitive techniques also help patients accept realistic, but less-than-desired, weight losses. Inappropriate feelings of failure after achieving modest but clinically important weight loss can lead to relapse and weight regain.

Behavioural therapy is an essential part of any successful weight management programme, which complements dietary and exercise therapy. Maintenance of weight loss after lifestyle modification, drug therapy, and weight loss surgery is more likely to depend on behaviour modification and continued support. Long-term behavioural therapy is more successful than short interventions. There are several ways in which behavioural therapy can be made available to individuals, such as specialist centres that include eating disorder and cognitive behaviour therapists, psychology clinics, self-help or commercial weight loss programmes, and internet-based programmes.

Drug treatment for obesity

Over the last few decades, numerous agents have been used to treat obesity. Most of these drugs are rarely used now, due to lack of efficacy or toxic side effects. Some drugs that have been used in the past are shown in *Table 4.8*. Some agents are approved by the US Food and Drug Administration (FDA) and European agencies only for short-term use. There is some evidence of their efficacy but very few data support their long-term benefits or improvements in comorbidities. Rimonabant, which is a CB_1 receptor antagonist, was approved for long-term use in Europe and was recently withdrawn due to an increased risk of psychiatric side effects. This highlights the need for strong long-term research data before approving weight loss agents and finding an appropriate agent with good efficacy and an acceptable side effect profile continues to be elusive. Newer therapeutic agents in development are discussed in Chapter 5.

Table 4.8 Pharmacological agents to treat obesity

Drugs approved for long-term use (12 months or more)
- Orlistat: intestinal lipase inhibitor (prescription or OTC – see main text opposite)

Licensed diabetes agents causing weight loss
- Metformin
- Pramlintide (amylin)
- GLP-1 analogues (exenatide, liraglutide)

Drugs (approved in some countries) for short-term use (up to 12 weeks)
- Phentermine
- Diethylpropion
- Benzphetamine
- Mazindol
- Phendimetrazine

Drugs recently withdrawn from use
- Sibutramine: Serotonin and noradrenaline reuptake inhibitor
- Rimonabant: Selective cannabinoid type CB_1 receptor antagonist

Drugs considered for weight management in the past (not recommended for routine use)
- Thyroid extract
- Amphetamines
- Dinitrophenol
- Aminoxaphen
- Ephedrine/Caffeine, ephedra alkaloids (ma huang)
- Digitalis/Diuretics
- Fenfluramine
- Dexfenfluramine
- Phenmetrazine
- Phenylpropanolamine
- Topiramate
- Zonisamide
- Fluoxetine
- Bupropion

Orlistat

- *Mechanism of action.* It inhibits pancreatic and intestinal lipases, resulting in inhibition of absorption of about 30% of dietary triglycerides. It is not absorbed systemically and does not affect systemic lipases (**4.8**).
- *Recommended dosage.* This is a dose of 120 mg three times daily (either with a meal or up to 1 hour after each meal) combined with lifestyle and behavioural therapy. A lower dose of 60 mg three times daily has recently been approved for 'over-the-counter' sales in many countries.
- *Indications.* Treatment of obesity when BMI >30 kg/m² or BMI >28 kg/m² with associated risk factors.
- *Contraindications.* Chronic malabsorption, cholestasis, breast-feeding, and hypersensitivity.
- *Adverse effects.* Gastrointestinal (GI) side effects such as oily spotting, flatus with discharge, faecal urgency, fatty or oily stool, increased defecation, and faecal incontinence. The absorption of fat-soluble vitamins and β-carotene may be impaired.
- *Recommendations.* Withdrawal rate due to GI side effects can be lowered by appropriate dietary advice; people should be advised to avoid high fat meals as the incidence of GI adverse events appears to be related to the dietary fat content. Patients should be encouraged to increase their intake of fruit and vegetables. The use of vitamin supplements should also be considered. Current evidence supports use for up to 48 months duration but may be considered for weight maintenance if there is a risk of weight regain on completion of therapy. Further research is required to support prolonged use.

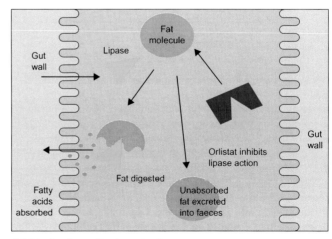

4.8 Mechanism of action of orlistat.

- *Use in children and adolescents.* The efficacy and safety profile appears to be similar in adolescents.
- *Efficacy.* Mean weight loss over placebo after 2 years of treatment = 3.5 kg (10.3 kg vs 6.1 kg); 5% weight loss achieved in 58% (vs 32%); 10% weight loss achieved in 39% (vs 18%) (**4.9, 4.10**). Modest reductions in several cardiovascular risk factors have been found, including total and low-density lipoprotein cholesterol (LDL-C), fasting insulin, and BP. Weight loss achieved in obese patients with diabetes is less than non-diabetes subjects but there is an approximately 0.4% reduction in HbA_{1c}. The 4-year XENDOS (XENical in the prevention of Diabetes in Obese Subjects) study showed some weight regain in both orlistat-treated and placebo groups but there was a significant reduction in the progression rates to type 2 diabetes (18.8% in the orlistat group vs 28.8%; relative risk reduction of 45%). In those who were known

to have impaired glucose tolerance at baseline there was 37% relative risk reduction in the development of type 2 diabetes.

Sibutramine

Sibutramine was withdrawn by the European Medicines Agency (EMA) in January 2010 and subsequently from the USA in October 2010. It was a centrally-acting inhibitor of both serotonin and noradrenaline reuptake with little effect on dopamine receptors. It limited food intake by enhancement of the natural satiety process. The starting dose was 10 mg/day, which could be increased to 15 mg/day if the weight loss achieved in 4 weeks was less than 2 kg. It was used with strict blood pressure and heart rate monitoring. Adverse effects were headache, dry mouth, anorexia, insomnia, constipation, hypertension, tachycardia and palpitations. Mean weight loss after 24 weeks of treatment was 1.2% with placebo, 6.1% with 10 mg/day and 7.4% with 15 mg/day (**4.11, 4.12**).

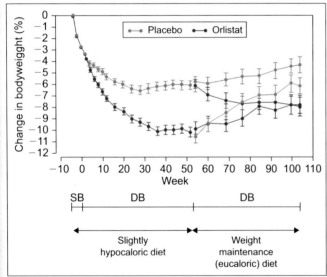

4.9 Weight loss with orlistat in a randomized, placebo-controlled trial over 2 years and prevention of weight regain in obese subjects. After a dietary lead-in period of 4 weeks, 688 patients were randomized to treatment with orlistat 120 mg three times daily or placebo for the first 12 months. A diet with 600 kcal/day deficit was recommended in the first year followed by a weight maintenance diet in the second year. After 12 months they were further randomized to orlistat or placebo. Patients who took orlistat in the initial 12 months lost an average of 10.3 kg in comparison with weight loss of 6.1 kg in the placebo group. There was less weight regain in patients who continued to take orlistat (with permission[7]). DB, double-blind, placebo-controlled treatment during years 1 and 2; SB, single-blind lead-in period of 4 weeks; error bars = standard error of the mean (SEM).

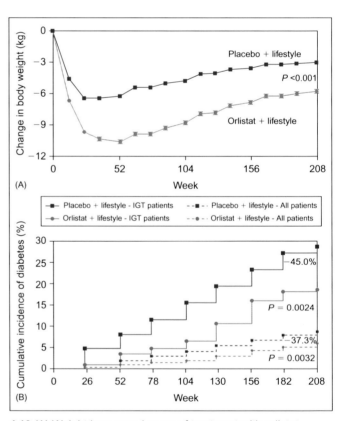

4.10 (A) Weight loss over 4 years of treatment with orlistat plus lifestyle or placebo plus lifestyle in obese patients and (B) diabetes prevention with orlistat in the XENDOS study (with permission[8]). IGT, impaired glucose tolerance.

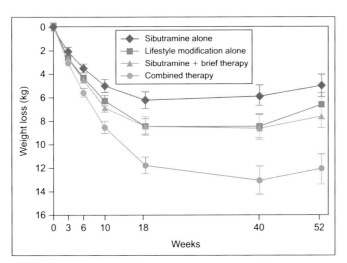

4.11 Weight loss with sibutramine when combined with lifestyle modification and behaviour therapy (with permission[9]). In this 1-year trial, 224 obese adults were randomly assigned to receive 15 mg of sibutramine/day alone (Group 1), lifestyle-modification counselling alone (Group 2), sibutramine plus lifestyle-modification counselling (i.e. combined therapy) (Group 3), or sibutramine plus a brief lifestyle-modification counselling (Group 4). All subjects were prescribed the same diet (1200–1500 kcal/day) and exercise regimen. At 1 year, subjects who received combined therapy lost a mean (±SD) of 12.1±9.8 kg, whereas those receiving sibutramine alone lost 5.0±7.4 kg, those treated by lifestyle modification alone lost 6.7±7.9 kg, and those receiving sibutramine plus brief therapy lost 7.5±8.0 kg ($P < 0.001$). This emphasizes the importance of prescribing weight-loss medications in combination with lifestyle modification and behaviour therapy.

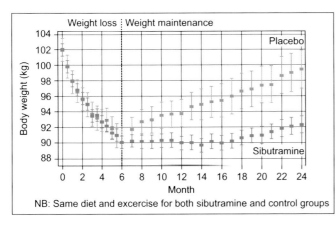

4.12 Effect of sibutramine on weight maintenance after initial weight loss—Sibutramine Trial of Obesity Reduction and Maintenance (STORM) study (with permission[10]).

Withdrawal of sibutramine – the SCOUT trial

The Sibutramine Cardiovascular Outcomes Study (SCOUT) was a randomised, double-blind, placebo-controlled study in 10 744 obese and overweight patients with cardiovascular disease and/or type 2 diabetes treated over a 6-year period (**4.13**). The results showed that these high-risk patients treated with sibutramine had a 16% increased risk of adverse events such as myocardial infarction, stroke, cardiac arrest and cardiovascular death compared with placebo-treated patients (11.4% vs 10.0%; hazard ratio 1.16 [95% CI 1.029–1.311]; $P = 0.016$).[9] The mean weight loss achieved with sibutramine in all clinical trials was modest, decreasing body weight by approximately 2–4 kg more than placebo, which may not be sustained after cessation of treatment. Although sibutramine was contraindicated in these high-risk patients as per the previous licence of use, it was felt that the risks of cardiovascular adverse events in the obese population outweighed the benefits and therefore sibutramine was withdrawn.

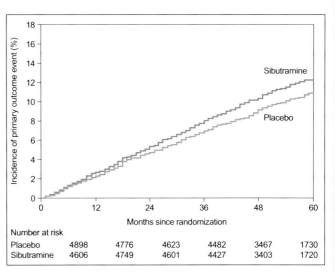

4.13 Effect of Sibutramine on Cardiovascular Outcomes in Overweight and Obese Subjects – the SCOUT trial. Kaplan–Meier plots of the incidence of a 'primary outcome event' according to the time from randomisation, which included non-fatal myocardial infarction, non-fatal stroke, resuscitation after cardiac arrest and cardiovascular death. The analyses were adjusted for age, sex (with male sex as the reference) and country. The risk of a primary outcome event was increased by 16% in the sibutramine group as compared with the placebo group ($P = 0.02$), with overall incidences of 11.4% and 10.0%, in the two groups (with permission[11]).

Rimonabant

Rimonabant was withdrawn from Europe in October 2008 and is not approved by the FDA. It was a selective cannabinoid type CB_1 receptor antagonist. It was thought to primarily regulate food intake via a centrally-mediated action in addition to peripheral metabolic effects. It was said to act on cannabinoid receptors in the brain, adipose tissue, liver, muscle and gastrointestinal tract. The recommended dosage was 20 mg once daily combined with lifestyle changes and behavioural therapy. It was contraindicated in people with a past history of depression and those taking antidepressant medication. Common adverse effects were upper respiratory tract infection, nausea, gastroenteritis, anxiety, insomnia, mood alterations, depressive disorders, sleep disorders, dizziness and memory loss. Subjects who experienced mood changes on treatment were advised to discontinue treatment immediately and seek medical advice. In addition to significant weight loss, there were improvements in glycaemic control and lipid profile. Data supporting the use of Rimonabant were obtained from the RIO-North America, RIO-Europe, RIO-Lipids, RIO-Diabetes and SERENADE studies (**4.14**).

Withdrawal of rimonabant

Comprehensive Rimonabant Evaluation Study of Cardiovascular Endpoints and Outcomes (CRESCENDO), a randomised, multicentre, placebo-controlled trial was prematurely discontinued because of concerns by health regulatory authorities in three countries about suicide in individuals receiving rimonabant. The composite primary endpoint of cardiovascular death, myocardial infarction or stroke occurred in 3.9% of patients assigned to rimonabant and 4.0% assigned to placebo (hazard ratio 0.97; 95% CI 0.84–1.12; $P = 0.68$). With rimonabant, gastrointestinal (33% vs 22%), neuropsychiatric (32% vs 21%) and serious psychiatric side-effects (2.5% vs 1.3%) were significantly increased compared with placebo. Four patients in the rimonabant group and one in the placebo group committed suicide.[12] Following concern expressed officially by the EMA in 2008, the drug manufacturer ceased marketing rimonabant in Europe because of psychiatric concerns that were emerging from post-marketing registries and ongoing clinical trials. In January 2009, the EMA withdrew altogether its marketing authorisation for rimonabant.

Future therapeutic targets and promising anti-obesity drugs in development are discussed in Chapter 5.

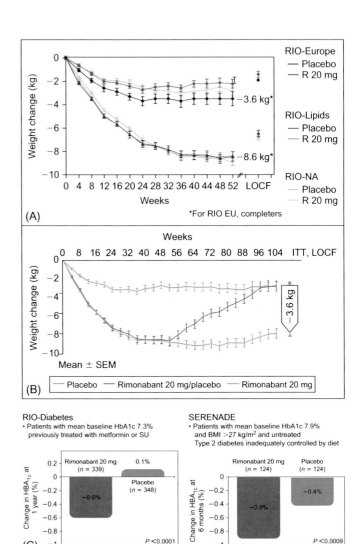

4.14 (A) Weight change with rimonabant: pooled data from RIO-Europe, RIO-Lipids, and RIO-North America.[13–15] (B) RIO-North America: prevention of weight regain with long-term rimonabant therapy.[14] (C) HbA$_{1c}$ change with rimonabant in RIO-Diabetes and SERENADE studies.[16,17]

Surgical treatment of obesity

Liposuction

Liposuction involves the removal of subcutaneous body fat by aspiration after injection of saline. It is performed as a cosmetic procedure, which causes a short-term reduction in fat mass and weight but does not appear to improve insulin sensitivity or cardiovascular risk factors. It is not recommended as a treatment option for obesity as no metabolic benefits are seen and the long-term consequences are unknown.

Bariatric surgery

Surgical treatments for obesity have been in constant development for more than 50 years but their use, until recently, has been very limited due to the risk of death and complications, their invasiveness, the costs involved, the need for intensive postoperative management, and a lack of long-term outcome and safety data. The surgical techniques used today are less complicated and the use of minimally invasive laparoscopic techniques has drastically cut down the incidence of perioperative complications. With improved surgical instruments and techniques, and an overall improvement in the standards of postoperative care, the field of bariatric surgery is gaining popularity (*Table 4.9*). We are beginning to see the long-term benefits of surgery and confidence in the safety profile of some procedures is improving. In the 1980s and 1990s there were numerous reports supporting the fact that, in addition to causing significant weight loss, bariatric surgery led to remission and improvement of various comorbidities (particularly type 2 diabetes). This created a lot of interest among health professionals and the popularity of surgical treatment for obesity has been on an upward trend ever since.

Older procedures (less common or not used today)
Jejuno-ileal bypass
This was one of the first bariatric procedures, used in the 1950s. The proximal jejunum was diverted to the distal part of the gut. As a long segment of small intestine was excluded, there was very limited absorption. Of the many variations that existed, one is shown in **4.15**. This procedure was very effective in causing sustained weight loss but its use was ultimately discontinued due to serious adverse effects such as offensive diarrhoea, electrolyte imbalances, renal (oxalate) calculi, progressive hepatic fibrosis, and eventually liver failure.

Open Roux-en-Y gastric bypass
This was introduced by Edward Mason in 1960. In this procedure, the stomach was reduced to a small upper gastric pouch, which drained into a Roux-en-Y limb of proximal jejunum (variable lengths used between 40 and 150 cm). It was designed as a combined malabsorptive and restrictive procedure. This procedure, although effective, was limited by significant perioperative mortality and complication rates for several decades. Several modifications have been

Table 4.9 Types of bariatric surgery

Mechanism of action	Common surgery types
Restrictive	Laparoscopic adjustable gastric banding Vertical banded gastroplasty
Malabsorptive	Biliopancreatic diversion: Scopinaro procedure Biliopancreatic diversion with duodenal switch
Combined	Roux-en-Y gastric bypass

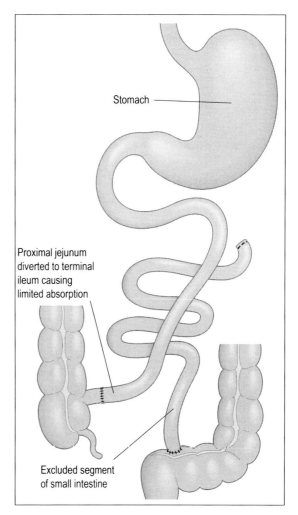

Stomach

Proximal jejunum diverted to terminal ileum causing limited absorption

Excluded segment of small intestine

4.15 Jejuno-ileal bypass.

tried over the years and this procedure is usually performed laparoscopically today.

Gastroplasty

In the 1970s, this purely restrictive procedure was introduced. It involved creating a small upper gastric pouch draining through a narrow stoma into the remainder of the stomach. It was less complicated than Roux-en-Y gastric bypass and several variations were introduced. In the 1980s, vertical banded gastroplasty (**4.16**) gained popularity, but evidence for the long-term efficacy of this procedure was disappointing. Gastric banding is now the most commonly performed restrictive procedure.

Open biliopancreatic diversion (4.17)

This was introduced by Nicolo Scopinaro in the 1970s. It involved distal, horizontal gastrectomy, leaving an upper gastric pouch of 200–500 ml, which was anastomosed to a 250 cm length of terminal ileum ('alimentary limb'). The 'biliopancreatic limb' was attached to the small intestine, 50 cm proximal to the ileocaecal valve. The 'common limb' (50 cm) was the only segment where bile and nutrients could mix, enabling the absorption of fat and starch. The non-caloric nutrients were absorbed in the alimentary limb (250 cm).

Intragastric balloon (IGB) (4.18)

A soft, saline-filled balloon is placed in the stomach endoscopically. It promotes satiety and causes restriction. It is still being used in several centres in Europe and South America. Although the risk of complications is lower than other surgical types, the weight loss achieved is transient and failure rates are high.

Commonly used procedures

Laparoscopic adjustable gastric band (4.19)

This was introduced in the mid-1990s. It is a restrictive procedure that involves placing an adjustable band in the upper part of the stomach, just distal to the gastro-oesophageal junction. The amount of restriction can be

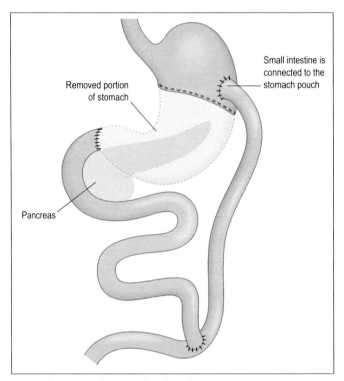

4.17 Biliopancreatic diversion: Scopinaro procedure.

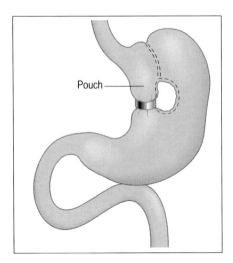

4.16 Vertical banded gastroplasty.

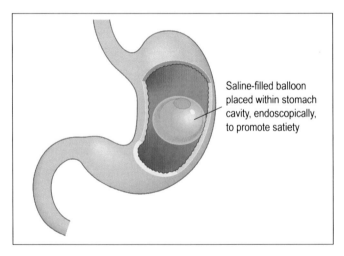

4.18 Intragastric balloon.

altered by injecting or withdrawing saline from the band through a subcutaneous port (similar to that used for long-term venous access for chemotherapy patients).

Laparoscopic Roux-en-Y gastric bypass (4.20)
This is the commonest procedure performed in the world today. The mortality and complication rates have reduced significantly since the use of minimally invasive techniques.

Laparoscopic biliopancreatic diversion
This is technically challenging and is best performed by surgeons who are experienced in this procedure and in centres where skilled multidisciplinary support is available.

Laparoscopic biliopancreatic diversion with duodenal switch (4.21)
In this procedure, a sleeve gastrectomy (SG) is performed (rather than the original horizontal gastrectomy in the Scopinaro type) leaving a gastric reservoir of 150–200 ml. The duodenum is closed about 2 cm distal to the pylorus and a duodeno-ileal anastomosis is performed. The gastric fundus is almost entirely resected, while the antrum, pylorus, and a short segment of duodenum are preserved along with the vagus nerve. Moreover, the 'common limb' is about 100 cm as opposed to 50 cm in the original procedure. This procedure can be done in two stages in very obese subjects (BMI >60 kg/m^2); initially a sleeve gastrectomy is performed to allow moderate weight loss.

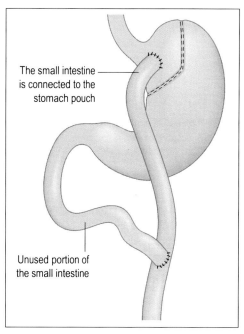

4.20 Roux-en-Y gastric bypass.

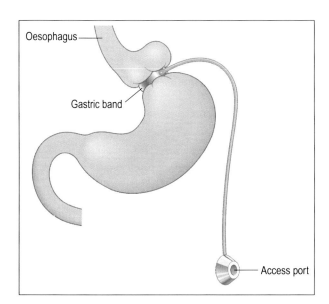

4.19 Laparoscopic adjustable gastric band.

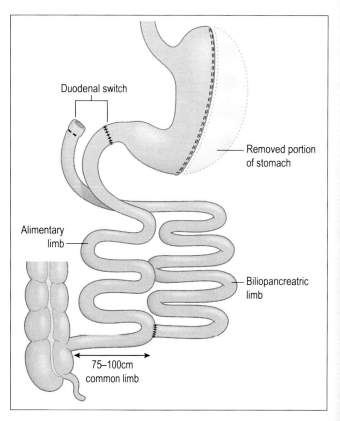

4.21 Biliopancreatic diversion with duodenal switch.

The rest of the procedure can be performed safely after a period of weight loss.

Newer surgical procedures and techniques

Newer procedures and techniques, such as duodenal-jejunal bypass (DJB), sleeve gastrectomy, ileal interposition (IT), mid-jejunal resection, omentectomy, robotic surgery, and endoluminal procedures (natural orifice transluminal endoscopic surgery (NOTES)), are discussed in more detail in Chapter 5.

Criteria for the surgical treatment of obesity

Several criteria for the surgical treatment of obesity exist worldwide. In most places, the choice of surgery is influenced by a person's ability to pay or the availability of health insurance cover. In public funded healthcare services like the NHS (UK), patient selection depends heavily on the availability of resources, of experienced surgeons and of bariatric units with a skilled multidisciplinary team. The main aim is to identify those subjects who are most likely to benefit from surgery (the risk of obesity and its complications versus the potential benefits of surgery) with acceptable perioperative risk.

- BMI >40 kg/m^2.
- BMI >35 kg/m^2 with serious obesity-related comorbidities that are likely to improve with surgery.
- Failed non-surgical attempts at weight loss such as supervised dietary and exercise programmes and a trial of anti-obesity drugs (often required to participate in a weight management programme in a specialized centre).
- Evaluated by an experienced bariatric surgeon.
- Fit for anaesthesia and surgery.
- Willingness to maintain long-term follow-up after surgery.
- Can be the first-line therapy for subjects with BMI >50 kg/m^2 if appropriate.

Preoperative evaluation and education

- Routine psychological evaluation should be encouraged to ensure that all aspects of the surgical procedure, risks, and post-procedure requirements are clearly understood.
- Surgery is not recommended in subjects with significant psychiatric illness, eating disorders, and behavioural problems.
- Surgical failure, weight regain, and complications after surgery should be discussed and steps should be taken to avoid these.

- Liaising with a multidisciplinary team is important before and after surgery.
- Patients should take responsibility (patient accountability) for lifestyle changes before and after surgery.

Advantages, disadvantages, and adverse effects associated with common bariatric procedures

Common perioperative complications after abdominal surgery include infection, haemorrhage, perforation, intestinal obstruction, hernia, and deep vein thrombosis (DVT).

Other adverse events are described for each surgical type as follows:

- Laparoscopic adjustable gastric banding (LAGB) (*Table 4.10*).
- Roux-en-Y gastric bypass (RYGB) (*Table 4.11*).
- Biliopancreatic diversion (BPD) (including duodenal switch (DS)) (*Table 4.12*).

Additional benefits of bariatric surgery (*Table 4.13*)

- Diabetes remission/improvement in glycaemic control.
- Improved BP control—evidence up to 2 years (but long-term results disappointing).
- Improvements in dyslipidaemia.
- Heart: ↓ left ventricular mass, ↑ ejection fraction, ↓ atherosclerosis, ↓myocardial infarction.
- Fertility: ↓ sex hormone-binding globulin, ↑ testosterone, ↑ oestrogen (no change in hirsutism), ↑ ovulation.
- ↓ Gestational diabetes mellitus (GDM), ↓ pre-eclampsia, ↓ lower segment Caesarean section (LSCS) rates, ↓ birth weight.
- ↓ Gastro-oesophageal reflux disease.
- ↓ Asthma.
- ↓ Cancers.
- ↓ Backache, arthritis.
- Improved liver profile (non-alcoholic steatohepatitis (NASH)).
- ↓ Incontinence problems.
- ↓ Pseudotumour cerebri.
- ↓ Venous stasis and ulcers.

Table 4.10 Laparoscopic adjustable gastric banding

Advantages	Disadvantages	Adverse effects
• Lower mortality rate • Technically less complicated • Fully reversible • Lower length of hospital stay • Shorter recovery • Adjustable restriction according to response • Nutritional deficiencies less common (no malabsorption)	• Not suitable for very obese • Less efficacy than others • High failure rate • Patient-dependent—diet, motivation • High incidence of minor complications • High reoperation rates • Gradual weight loss (variable) • Slow improvement/changes in comorbidities requiring constant monitoring • Long-term follow-up required • Skilled personnel to adjust band and diet advice	• Nausea, vomiting, reflux • Stoma obstruction, dysphagia • Altered bowel habits • Band dislocation/slippage • Oesophageal dysmotility/dilatation • Band migration/erosion • Band/port leakage • Band malfunction • Port displacement • Port site discomfort, infection

Table 4.11 Roux-en-Y gastric bypass

Advantages	Disadvantages	Adverse effects
• Significant excess weight loss (more than laparoscopic adjustable gastric banding) • Remission/improvement of comorbidities particularly diabetes • Less complication/mortality than biliopancreatic diversion	• Irreversible • Restricted intake (volume) • Higher adverse effects • Need for long-term monitoring • Risk of weight regain • Nutritional deficiencies	• Hernia • Anastomotic leakage • Stomal ulcers, stricture, obstruction • Nausea, vomiting • Dumping syndrome • Iron, B12, vitamin D deficiency

Table 4.12 Biliopancreatic diversion (including duodenal switch)

Advantages	Disadvantages	Adverse effects
• Less diet restriction than bypass • Less risk of dumping • Significant excess weight loss (more than others) • Remission/improvement of comorbidities particularly diabetes • Low risk of weight regain • Can be performed in two stages	• Irreversible • Complicated procedure • Highest complication rate/ mortality • Serious protein malnutrition • Nutritional deficiencies • Requires long-term intensive monitoring	• Hernia • Anastomotic leakage • Stomal ulcers, stricture, obstruction • Nausea, vomiting • Bloating, flatulence, loose stools • Protein malnutrition • Vitamin and mineral deficiencies

Table 4.13 Summary of weight loss outcomes, mortality rate and diabetes remission rate after common bariatric procedures.[18,19]

Procedure	Excess weight loss (%)	Diabetes remission rate (%)	Mortality (%) <30 days	Mortality (%) >30 days to 2 years
LAGB	46.2	56.7	O = 0.18 L = 0.06	O = 0.00 L = 0.00
Gastroplasty	55.5	79.7	O = 0.33 L = 0.21	O = 0.23 L = 0.00
RYGB	59.7	80.3	O = 0.44 L = 0.16	O = 0.69 L = 0.09
BPD and DS	63.6	95.1	O = 0.76 L = 1.11	O = 0.85 L = NA
All procedures	55.9	78.1	0.28	0.35

L = laparoscopic; O = open.

- Pickwickian syndrome, hypoventilation, obstructive sleep apnoea syndrome (OSAS)—reduced need for non-invasive ventilation.
- Improved quality of life (Short-Form 36), employment.
- ↓ Depression.

Mortality risk and prognosis after various bariatric procedures

Table 4.13 summarises the average excess weight loss achieved after common surgical procedures based on large meta-analyses.[16, 17] *Table 4.13* also highlights the diabetes remission rate, which is more impressive after malabsorptive procedures. It is worth noting that, after malabsorptive procedures, improvements in glycaemic control occur within hours and days of surgery, before any meaningful weight loss can occur. It is therefore acknowledged that diabetes remission after malabsorptive surgery occurs due to a variety of mechanisms, independent of weight loss, which are beyond the scope of this book. However, malabsorptive procedures also carry a higher risk of mortality. The choice of bariatric procedure in an individual has to be based on the degree of weight loss desired, the presence of comorbidities

such as type 2 diabetes and the operative risk for the individual concerned (**4.22**).

The prospective, controlled Swedish Obese Subjects study[18] involved 4047 obese subjects. 2010 underwent bariatric surgery (surgery group) and 2037 received conventional treatment (matched control group) (**4.23**). The average weight change in control subjects was not significant (less than ±2%) during the recording period of up to 15 years. Maximum weight losses in the surgical subgroups were observed after 1–2 years: gastric bypass, 32%; vertical-banded gastroplasty, 25%; and banding, 20%. After 10 years, the weight losses from baseline were stabilized at 25%, 16%, and 14%, respectively. There were 129 deaths in the control group and 101 deaths in the surgery group. The unadjusted overall hazard ratio was 0.76 in the surgery group ($P = 0.04$), as compared with the control group, and the hazard ratio adjusted for sex, age, and risk factors was 0.71 ($P = 0.01$).

In a large retrospective cohort study,[19] long-term mortality was determined among 9949 patients who had undergone gastric bypass surgery and 9628 severely obese persons who had applied for driver's licenses between 1984 and 2002 (**4.24**). Of these subjects, 7925 surgical patients and 7925 severely obese control subjects were matched for age, sex, and BMI. During a mean follow-up of 7.1 years, adjusted long-term mortality from any cause in the

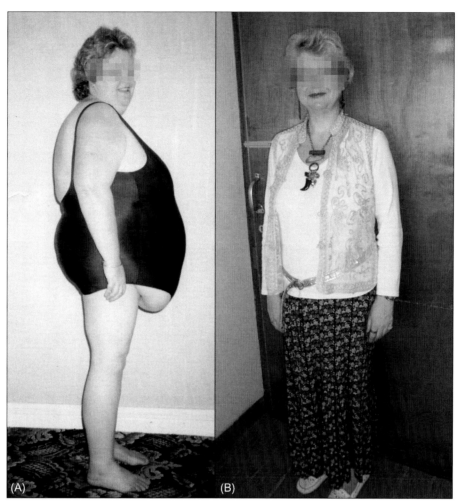

4.22 Photographs of a patient (A) before and (B) 2 years after duodenal switch (BMI improved from 51 to 27 with significant improvements in comorbidities and activities of daily living).

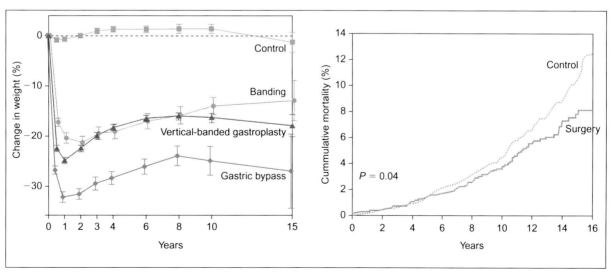

4.23 Effects of bariatric surgery on mortality in Swedish obese subjects. (A) Mean percentage weight change during a 15-year period in the control group and the surgery group. (B) Unadjusted cumulative mortality (with permission[20]).

4.24 Long-term mortality after gastric bypass surgery—survival according to BMI in the surgery group and the control group (with permission[21]).

surgery group decreased by 40%, as compared with that in the control group (37.6 vs 57.1 deaths per 10 000 person-years; $P < 0.001$); cause-specific mortality in the surgery group decreased by 56% for coronary artery disease (2.6 vs 5.9 per 10 000 person-years; $P = 0.006$), by 92% for diabetes (0.4 vs 3.4 per 10 000 person-years; $P = 0.005$), and by 60% for cancer (5.5 vs 13.3 per 10 000 person-years; $P < 0.001$).

In summary, the choice of anti-obesity treatment depends on a thorough assessment of an individual's problems. The presence of comorbidities and obesity-induced complications, an individual's motivation and willingness to change and their past experiences and suitability for drug/surgical therapy tend to determine the level of intervention. Availability of specialist services and the costs involved are likely to influence the choice of surgical treatment in most parts of the world. Lifestyle changes and behavioural therapy should be the first step before considering drugs or surgical procedures. Patient education regarding benefits of therapy (as compared with expectations) and risks will improve compliance. A detailed management plan needs to include weight maintenance strategies (after initial weight loss) for successful treatment of obesity in the long term.

References

1. Kopelman PG, Caterson ID, Dietz WH. *Clinical Obesity in Adults and Children*, 3rd edn. Chichester: Wiley–Blackwell; 2009.
2. Flechtner-Mors M, Ditschuneit HH, Johnson TD, Suchard MA, Adler G. Metabolic and weight loss effects of long-term dietary intervention in obese patients: four-year results. *Obesity* 2000; **8**: 399–402.
3. Paisey RB, Frost J, Harvey P, *et al.* Five year results of a prospective very low calorie diet or conventional weight loss programme in type 2 diabetes. *J Hum Nutr Diet* 2002; **15**: 121–7.
4. Tremblay A, Despres JP, Maheux J, *et al.* Normalization of the metabolic profile in obese women by exercise and a low fat diet. *Med Sci Sports Exerc* 1991; **23**: 1326–31.
5. Sandvik L, Erikssen J, Thaulow E, *et al.* Physical fitness as a predictor of mortality among healthy, middle-aged Norwegian men. *N Engl J Med* 1993; **328**: 533–7.

6. Wadden TA, Foster GD. Behavioral treatment of obesity. *Med Clin North Am* 2000; **84**: 441–61, vii.

7. Sjostrom L, Rissanen A, Andersen T, *et al.* Randomised placebo-controlled trial of orlistat for weight loss and prevention of weight regain in obese patients. European Multicentre Orlistat Study Group. *Lancet* 1998; **352**: 167–72.

8. Torgerson JS, Hauptman J, Boldrin MN, Sjostrom L. XENical in the Prevention of Diabetes in Obese Subjects (XENDOS) study: a randomized study of orlistat as an adjunct to lifestyle changes for the prevention of type 2 diabetes in obese patients. *Diabetes Care* 2004; **27**: 155–61.

9. Wadden TA, Berkowitz RI, Womble LG, *et al.* Randomized trial of lifestyle modification and pharmacotherapy for obesity. *N Engl J Med* 2005; **353**: 2111–20.

10. James WP, Astrup A, Finer N, *et al.* Effect of sibutramine on weight maintenance after weight loss: a randomised trial. STORM Study Group. Sibutramine Trial of Obesity Reduction and Maintenance. *Lancet* 2000; **356**: 2119–25.

11. James WP, Caterson ID, Coutinho W, *et al.* Effect of sibutramine on cardiovascular outcomes in overweight and obese subjects. *N Engl J Med* 2010; **363**: 905–17.

12. Topol EJ, Bousser MG, Fox KA, *et al.* Rimonabant for prevention of cardiovascular events (CRESCENDO): a randomised, multicentre, placebo-controlled trial. *Lancet* 2010; **376**: 517–23.

13. Van Gaal LF, Rissanen AM, Scheen AJ, Ziegler O, Rossner S. Effects of the cannabinoid-1 receptor blocker rimonabant on weight reduction and cardiovascular risk factors in overweight patients: 1-year experience from the RIO-Europe study. *Lancet* 2005; **365**: 1389–97.

14. Pi-Sunyer FX, Aronne LJ, Heshmati HM, Devin J, Rosenstock J. Effect of rimonabant, a cannabinoid-1 receptor blocker, on weight and cardiometabolic risk factors in overweight or obese patients: RIO-North America: a randomized controlled trial. *JAMA* 2006; **295**: 761–75.

15. Despres JP, Golay A, Sjostrom L. Effects of rimonabant on metabolic risk factors in overweight patients with dyslipidemia. *N Engl J Med* 2005; **353**: 2121–34.

16. Scheen AJ, Finer N, Hollander P, Jensen MD, Van Gaal LF. Efficacy and tolerability of rimonabant in overweight or obese patients with type 2 diabetes: a randomised controlled study. *Lancet* 2006; **368**: 1660–72.

17. Rosenstock J, Hollander P, Chevalier S, Iranmanesh A. SERENADE: the Study Evaluating Rimonabant Efficacy in Drug-Naive Diabetic Patients: effects of monotherapy with rimonabant, the first selective CB1 receptor antagonist, on glycemic control, body weight, and lipid profile in drug-naive type 2 diabetes. *Diabetes Care* 2008; **31**: 2169–76.

18. Buchwald H, Estok R, Fahrbach K, *et al.* Weight and type 2 diabetes after bariatric surgery: systematic review and meta-analysis. *Am J Med* 2009; **122**: 248–56.

19. Buchwald H, Estok R, Fahrbach K, Banel D, Sledge I. Trends in mortality in bariatric surgery: a systematic review and meta-analysis. *Surgery* 2007; **142**: 621–32.

20. Sjostrom L, Narbro K, Sjostrom CD, *et al.* Effects of bariatric surgery on mortality in Swedish obese subjects. *N Engl J Med* 2007; **357**: 741–52.

21. Adams TD, Gress RE, Smith SC, *et al.* Long-term mortality after gastric bypass surgery. *N Engl J Med* 2007; **357**: 753–61.

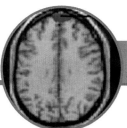

Chapter 5

Miscellaneous

Effective care of very obese subjects: barriers and solutions

The prevalence of obesity is increasing world-wide. The obese population is more prone to serious health problems that need specialized and hospital care. Hospitals and healthcare teams are therefore beginning to deal with larger and heavier patients, who are more likely to suffer from complex illnesses. They are more likely to be dependent in activities of daily living partly due to decreased mobility, require the skills of specialized multidisciplinary teams, and they tend to have longer stay in hospital. There need to be effective and planned strategies in place to be able to care for extremely obese people in order to minimize the risk of complications and injuries to the patients as well as the healthcare staff. Some barriers to effective care, and possible solutions, are summarized below.

Barriers to effective care of obesity

1. *Environmental factors predisposing to obesity*
   - Availability of excess, low-cost, high-calorie, and high-fat diet.
   - Dependence on transport and labour-saving devices.
   - Sedentary lifestyle.
   - Media hype and 'mixed' messages.
2. *Personal factors*
   - Denial and lack of self-responsibility.
   - Behavioural changes.
   - Optimistic bias and self-deception.
   - Lack of knowledge and coping strategies.
   - Reliance on 'crash diets' and 'quick fixes' rather than long-term lifestyle changes.
3. *Healthcare policy makers*
   - Lack of awareness and acknowledgement of obesity as a health risk.

- Lack of research into causes (e.g. genetic and lifestyle), behavioural influences, and management strategies.
- Limited resources and manpower.
- Lack of strategies and planning in identifying and targeting the high-risk population (e.g. children and adolescents).
- Will to promote long-term lifestyle changes in the community.

4. *Hospitals and healthcare providers*
   - Prejudice and discrimination of obese subjects.
   - Lack of specialized units for medical and surgical management of obesity.
   - Lack of awareness and knowledge.
   - Mistrust, misunderstanding, and legal claims.
   - Lack of planning and policies.
   - Caregiver injury and sickness absences.
   - Increased demand on resources and personnel to provide effective care.
   - Increased risk of complications and injuries to obese patients.
   - Lack of intensive care and postoperative care facilities suited to very obese patients.
   - Lack of equipment and health aids suitable for bariatric patients.
   - Need for a specialized multidisciplinary team approach (e.g. specialist nurses, occupational therapists, dietitians, behavioural therapists, postoperative management teams, manual handling experts, social services, etc.).

Priorities for effective care of very heavy subjects

1. *General*
   - Acknowledging obesity prevention as an important part of healthcare policy.

- Promotion of traditional healthy diet and daily physical exercise.
- Educational programmes targeting the 'at-risk' population.
- Targeting children and adolescents (e.g. school and community policies).
- Advertisements and media responsibility.
- Promoting medical research in this field.

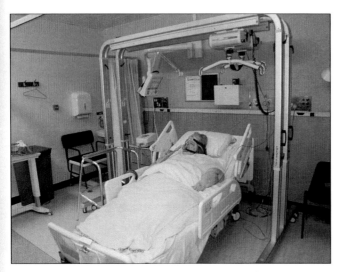

5.1 Very obese patient requiring hospital care. Hospitals need to be able to provide high-quality care by ensuring adequate availability of equipment such as heavy duty beds, hoists, and mobility aids. The safety of very heavy patients and the healthcare staff looking after them can be ensured by putting appropriate manual handling, transfer, and general healthcare policies in place.

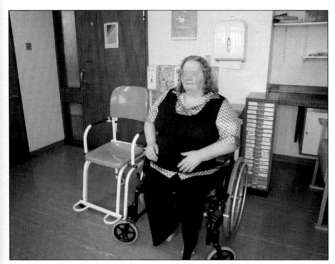

5.2 Simple factors such as a lack of appropriate wheelchairs, scales, and staff trained in manual handling procedures can often result in serious deficiencies in adequate and safe care of very heavy patients.

2. *Hospitals and healthcare providers* (**5.1, 5.2**)
   - Education of staff to improve awareness and minimize discrimination.
   - Establishment of centres that specialize in the medical and surgical management of obesity and related conditions.
   - Planning and availability of guidelines and policies for safe and effective management of bariatric subjects (e.g. manual handling, transfers, etc.).
   - Access to specialized centres that are able to provide intensive care and postoperative care to very obese subjects.
   - Availability of specialized multidisciplinary teams (e.g. dietitians, physiotherapist, occupational therapists, etc.).
   - Availability of medical equipment and health aids suitable for very obese subjects.

The future of obesity management

Obesity is now being recognized as an important and preventable health risk. Governments, health policy makers, and medical organizations are beginning to recognize the consequences of obesity and the benefits of weight loss. Several programmes have been planned to raise awareness about obesity at various levels; equal importance is given to the prevention of obesity in the population and management of the disease and its complications. Scientific research is encouraged to understand the reasons behind the obesity 'epidemic'. There is an urgent need to find treatments that are both efficient and safe. Some of the significant advances in this field are summarized in the following section.

Advances in pharmacotherapy
The following are some of the novel anti-obesity agents that are in different stages of development. The results of some of these drugs are very promising and hopefully we may see an increase in the number of anti-obesity pharmaceutical agents available to us in the next few years. Recent adverse experiences with anti-obesity drugs have highlighted the need for stricter scrutiny of the risk–benefit profile of these agents.

- *Cetilistat.* A novel lipase inhibitor that acts in the same way as orlistat by inhibiting pancreatic lipase. The efficacy is similar to orlistat but is thought to cause less gastrointestinal side effects. It has completed Phase 1 and 2 trials, which were encouraging with regards to better tolerability and is currently in Phase 3 trials.

- *Serotonin/noradrenaline reuptake inhibitors.*
  - *Tesofensine.* Dopamine, serotonin, and noradrenaline reuptake (triple) inhibitor thought to have less cardiovascular side effects than previous agents. Phase 2 trial results are encouraging.
  - *PSN 602.* 5-HT1A receptor agonist and monoamine reuptake inhibitor thought to have less cardiovascular side effects.
  - *Lorcaserin.* 5-HT2C receptor agonist that decreases food intake by targeting specific receptors in the brain without the cardiovascular side effects of previous agents. It failed to get FDA approval in 2010 based on available risk–benefit data.
  - *BVT 74316* and *PRX-07034.* 5-HT6 receptor antagonists that decrease food intake by enhancing satiety.
- *Novel cannabinoid (CB$_1$) receptor antagonists* (e.g. taranabant, CP-945, 598, AVE 1625, SLV 319). These agents are in different stages of development. It remains to be seen if the risk of psychiatric side effects are lower than in rimonabant. Prospects are poor unless a peripherally acting agent can be developed that does not cause central nervous system side effects.
- *Neuropeptide receptor ligands*
  - *Pramlintide.* Synthetic analogue of human amylin approved by the FDA for use in conjunction with insulin therapy in patients with type 1 or 2 diabetes. It delays gastric emptying, promotes satiety via hypothalamic receptors [different receptors than for glucagon-like peptide-1 (GLP-1)] and inhibits glucagon release. It is being studied in combination with other agents such as leptin, phentermine, and sibutramine. The results of pramlintide and metreleptin combination are encouraging.
  - *AC162352* (injectable) and *nasal spray (Nastech).* Synthetic analogues of human peptide YY (PYY 3-36), which decrease appetite and increase satiety.
  - *S-2367.* Selective neuropeptide Y5 receptor antagonist, which increases energy consumption, suppresses visceral fat accumulation, and improves blood glucose.
  - *Obinepitide.* Dual neuropeptide Y2–Y4 receptor agonist.
  - *TM30339.* Selective neuropeptide Y4 agonist.
  - *NGD-4715.* Melanin-concentrating hormone MCH-1 receptor antagonist.
- *Synthetic leptin.* An orally available leptin analogue that crosses the blood–brain barrier. It is also being studied in combination with other agents such as synthetic amylin and sibutramine.

- *Contrave.* A combination of bupropion (dopamine and noradrenaline reuptake inhibitor) and naltrexone (opioid receptor antagonist) enhances the release of α-melanocyte-stimulating hormone (α-MSH) and cocaine and amphetamine-regulated transcript (CART). It has a unique mechanism of action that works at two levels within the central nervous system: one associated with controlling the balance of food intake and metabolism and another involved in controlling food preference, reward, and cravings. Both drugs have individually shown some evidence of effectiveness in weight loss, and the combination is thought to have a synergistic effect. In December 2010 the FDA Drugs Advisory Committee recommended approval for this drug and the conduct of a post-marketing cardiovascular outcomes study.
- *Excalia.* A combination of bupropion and zonisamide (anticonvulsant) that enhances the release of α-MSH and CART and increases serotonin levels.
- *Qnexa.* A combination of phentermine (catecholamine releaser) and topiramate (anticonvulsant). Weight loss results are encouraging but this drug was unsuccessful in obtaining FDA approval in 2010 due to the high incidence of central nervous system and cardiac side effects.
- *Oxyntomodulin.* Decreases energy intake and increases energy expenditure by activation of GLP-1 receptors. Animal data and early human data show reduction in energy intake and reduced hunger with some weight loss.
- *Liraglutide.* A long-acting synthetic GLP-1 analogue has been shown to cause weight loss even in the absence of type 2 diabetes. In a double-blind, placebo-controlled 20-week trial, with open-label orlistat comparator, participants on liraglutide lost significantly more weight than did those on placebo or orlistat. Liraglutide reduced blood pressure and the prevalence of prediabetes.[1] Nausea and vomiting occurred more often in individuals on liraglutide than in those on placebo, but adverse events were mainly transient and rarely led to discontinuation of treatment.
- *β3-Adrenergic receptor agonists.* These increase energy expenditure by lipolysis and increase in thermogenesis.
- *KB5359.* A selective thyroid hormone receptor modulator.

Newer surgical procedures and techniques
Duodenal–jejunal bypass (5.3)
This was developed as an experimental antidiabetic procedure. The proximal duodenum is anastomosed to the

distal portion of small intestine (duodeno-jejunal type) or a pre-pyloric gastro-jejunostomy is performed. Long-term data are not yet available, but there appears to be significant remission/improvement of type 2 diabetes in addition to weight loss.

Sleeve gastrectomy (5.4)

This is usually performed as the first stage of a two-stage procedure in very obese patients (body mass index >60 kg/m²) or those with a high risk of mortality. After some weight loss, patients are able to have either a duodenal switch procedure or even a Roux-en-Y gastric bypass. This has been proposed as an independent anti-obesity procedure in its own right, particularly in very heavy patients or those with a high risk of perioperative complications. Further data to support this claim are awaited.

Ileal interposition/ileal transposition (5.5)

A small segment of ileum with its vascular and nerve supply intact is surgically interposed into the proximal small intestine, which leads to an increased exposure of the ileum to nutrients. This leads to exaggerated GLP-1 and peptide YY (PYY) responses to nutrients, resulting in reduced food intake, weight loss, and improved glucose homeostasis.

Mid-jejunal resection and omentectomy

These are experimental procedures that are promising in the short term, but further long-term data are awaited. They appear to be more efficient in improving the metabolic consequences of obesity rather than causing significant weight loss.

Robotic surgery

Primary and revisional bariatric surgery can be performed with the help of robotic assisted systems (e.g. daVinci robot system). These help the surgeon to increase precision and improve the outcomes of complex procedures. They are shown to be 30% faster than even experienced laparoscopic surgeons.[2]

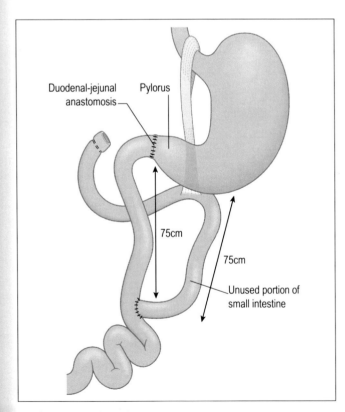

5.3 Duodenal–jejunal bypass.

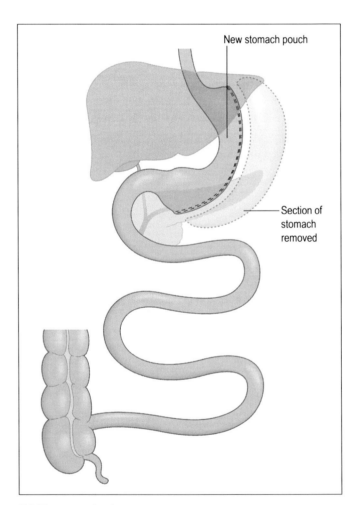

5.4 Sleeve gastrectomy.

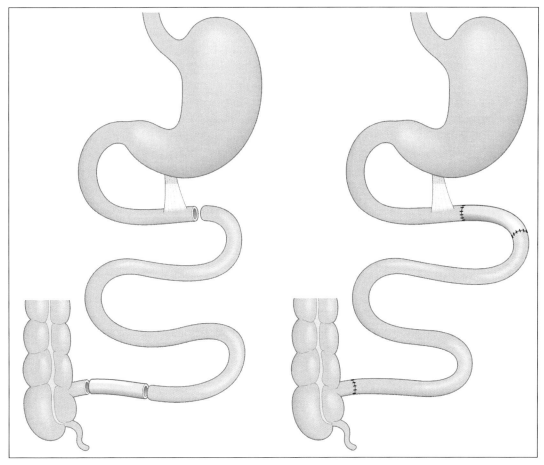

5.5 Ileal interposition/ileal transposition. A 10–20 cm portion of intact ileum (blue) is transposed into the proximal region of the small intestine, causing increased exposure to nutrients.

Endoluminal procedures (natural orifice transluminal endoscopic surgery)

These are procedures performed via 'natural orifices', reducing perioperative risk and mortality. Several restrictive (e.g. endoscopically inserted intragastric balloon, intraluminal gastric partitioning techniques) and malabsorptive procedures (e.g. polyethylene endoluminal duodeno-jejunal tube (EDJT)) are currently being studied in an attempt to develop a procedure that is safe as well as effective.

Advances in genetic research

For nearly two decades, epidemiological approaches to identify genetic causes for obesity were limited to candidate gene and genome-wide linkage studies. Although these techniques provided some valuable insight into the heritable causes of obesity and adiposity, progress has been painfully slow. The latest advances in the identification of genetic variations associated with chronic health problems using genome-wide association techniques have revived the initial optimism.

1. *Candidate gene studies*. Genes thought to be involved in the pathogenesis of obesity are identified and genetic variations at these loci are tested for association at the population level. Previous studies have been unable to demonstrate strong associations due to small sample sizes. The focus now is to perform association studies on large populations. For example, genetic variations in the *MC4R* (melanocortin-4 receptor) gene have been shown to be strongly associated with the risk of obesity.
2. *Genome-wide linkage studies*. This is a hypothesis-generating approach that examines the whole genome to identify the location of new genes for a particular disease. Populations

of related individuals such as siblings and/or nuclear families are studied to identify certain chromosomal locations related to a phenotype. When strong evidence of linkage is found, the region is screened further to identify the gene that contributes to variation in the phenotype. This method is successful for Mendelian disorders and diseases with large genetic effects, but is limited in the identification of continuous traits such as obesity. Although more than 250 human obesity quantitative trait loci have been identified, a recent meta-analysis of 37 genome-wide linkage studies could not identify a single obesity locus unequivocally.

3. *Genome-wide association studies.* This is the latest epidemiological gene finding technique. It involves screening of the whole genome to identify new and unanticipated genetic variations in large cohorts that may be associated with disease. Several discoveries have been made in the genetic associations of diabetes (type 1 and 2), prostate and breast cancer, Crohn's disease, rheumatoid arthritis, and multiple sclerosis using this new tool. Single nucleotide polymorphism (SNP) chips can identify more than 80% of the common genetic variations reported in the reference sequence of the human genome (International HapMap). Discovery of variations in the *FTO* gene and *INSIG2* gene associated with risk of weight gain (*see* Chapter 3) are some significant achievements in understanding the genomics of obesity using this technique.

There are several centres dedicated to identifying new genetic variants for obesity-related traits by combining data from several large-scale studies (e.g. GIANT—the Genetic Investigation of Anthropometric Traits Consortium, Wellcome Trust Case Control Consortium). Following the identification of these variants, there need to be extensive molecular and physiological studies to explore the underlying mechanisms and pathways that lead to clinical obesity.

Advances in treatment strategies: pharmacogenetics

Further advances in genetic screening and an understanding of how common genetic variation influences predisposition to, and the treatment of, obesity and associated metabolic diseases will lead to the individualization of obesity treatment and the establishment of appropriate targets. An example of how pharmacogenetics could lead to the identification of people likely to respond to a particular treatment is shown in **5.6**.

Functional neuro-imaging in obesity research

Until some years ago, the neuro-anatomical correlates of human feeding behaviour had remained largely unknown. With the introduction of functional neuro-imaging using positron emission tomography (PET) scans, functional MRI (fMRI) and manganese-enhanced fMRI in research, we are beginning to understand the role of different areas of the brain along with the associated physiological and biochemical processes involved in appetite and feeding regulation. PET scans measure the regional cerebral blood flow (rCBF) with the help of radio-labelled isotopes (^{15}O, ^{11}C, or ^{18}F), whereas fMRI measures changes in the blood oxygen level-dependent (BOLD) signal, which reflects concentrations of deoxyhaemoglobin, an intrinsic paramagnetic contrast agent. MRI-based techniques are better in describing the time course of brain events that control eating and provide the most precise map of where these events occur in the brain.

The hypothalamus and brainstem are thought to be the principal homeostatic brain areas responsible for regulating body weight. In the current obesogenic environment, food intake is largely determined by non-homeostatic factors, including cognition, emotion, and reward. These are primarily processed in cortico-limbic and higher cortical brain regions. The prefrontal cortex is associated with the cognitive control of feeding behaviour whereas the limbic areas (hippocampus, amygdala, anterior thalamic nuclei) and paralimbic areas (parahippocampal gyri, cingulate gyri, insula, caudal orbitofrontal cortex (OFC)) are associated with the processing and regulation of emotion, memory, olfaction, and behaviour. These form a multimodal area where sensory and visceral inputs elicited by food ingestion converge and are decoded in their reward value.

Significant differences have been shown in the brain responses to satiation in lean and obese individuals using these techniques (**5.7**).[4] Brain response to visual images of high and low calorie foods also appears to be different.[5] In response to images of high calorie foods, obese subjects when compared with normal weight controls, exhibited greater activation in a large number of regions hypothesized to mediate the motivational effects of food cues, indicating a hyperactive reward system in obese individuals.[6] In Prader–Willi syndrome there appears to be dysfunction of the satiety system and enhanced activation of the reward-mediating areas. Studies in leptin-deficient subjects following leptin replacement have shown that leptin acts on neural circuits, governing food intake to diminish the perception of food

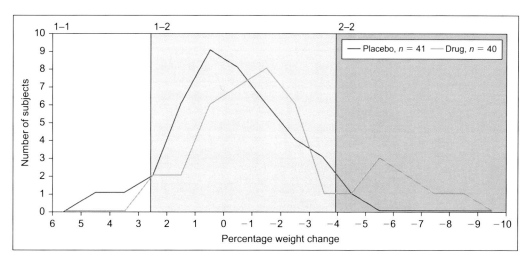

5.6 Graph showing the use of pharmacogenetics to evaluate efficacy of anti-obesity agent (with permission[3]). This graph illustrates the results of a small double-blind phase IIA efficacy clinical trial of a molecule intended for the treatment of obesity. Weight change in the 40 drug-treated patients (orange line) is compared with 41 placebo-treated patients (pink line) during the 2-month double-blind trial. There is an obvious hyper-responder subgroup in the treated patients, with patients losing as much as 9% weight during the trial. Two SNPs from two candidate genes are related to the proposed mechanism of action of this molecule, and one SNP from another candidate gene is thought to be implicated in theories of obesity, segregated with the hyper-responders. Each hyper-responder was homozygous for a single allele (labelled 2-2; dark green shaded section of the graph) with patients on the left side of the curves being more likely to be 1-1 homozygous (yellow shaded section). Heterozygous patients (1-2; light green section) clustered in the middle. In this experiment, treated patients with the 2-2 genotype for any of the three SNPs on average lost ~3.3 kg, whereas treated patients with the 1-1 genotype gained an average of ~1.3 kg. This pattern reassures us that the molecule has efficacy and that subsequent phase IIB trials might be enriched by using only patients who are 1-2 heterozygous and 2-2 homozygous, with the exclusion of 1-1 homozygous patients. In addition, although the 1-1 subgroup might be less responsive to this specific treatment, this subgroup could be used in clinical trials of other obesity drug candidates, which might subsequently allow a drug to be developed that is complementary to the first. *n*, total number of patients in study group.

reward while enhancing the response to satiety signals generated during food consumption.

Functional neuro-imaging has helped us to study brain function *in vivo* and non-invasively. It has helped to unravel the role of the reward system in the control of feeding behaviour and has highlighted the importance of non-homeostatic factors such as cognition, emotion, and other food-related stimuli. New combined methods and behavioural paradigms may help us to gain further insight into the pathophysiology of abnormal eating behaviour and obesity. These techniques may be useful in determining whether pharmacological or other interventions have an impact on appropriate neuronal substrates and could be used to predict the efficacy of such intervention.

Obesity prevention

Obesity is associated with serious comorbidities and health risks. In addition to causing physical illnesses and disabilities, obesity has a significant impact on social well-being and quality of life. Over the last few decades, some progress has been made in identifying effective interventions to reduce obesity and in improving obesity-related comorbidities. As obesity has reached epidemic proportions, we need to focus on population-based strategies to prevent weight gain and improve the social and physical environments to promote healthy eating and increased physical activity.[7,8] Population-based approaches to obesity prevention are complementary to clinical preventive and obesity management strategies. Several healthcare planning bodies have realized the need to prioritize population-based obesity prevention policies to target adults as well as children.

Individual

1. Maintaining energy balance (dietary changes and increased physical activity) by focusing on long-term behavioural changes using self-monitoring, goal-setting and problem-solving techniques.

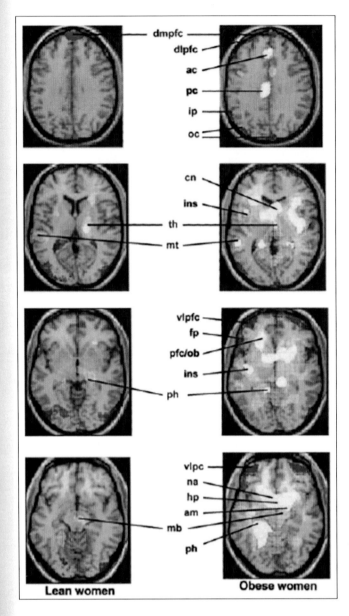

5.7 Effect of satiation on brain activity in obese and lean women (with permission[4]). Twelve obese women (body mass index >35) and 10 lean healthy women were studied after 36-hour fasts and liquid formula meals. Brain regions with significant increases in cerebral blood flow (CBF) in response to satiation are shown in blue; brain regions with significant decreases in CBF in response to satiation are shown in yellow. Satiation produced significant increases in CBF in the prefrontal cortex (pfc) and significant decreases in thalamus, insular cortex, para-hippocampal gyrus, temporal cortex and cerebellum, hypothalamus, cingulate, nucleus accumbens, and amygdala. Compared with lean women, obese women had significantly greater increases in CBF in the prefrontal cortex and greater decreases in CBF in paralimbic areas. Dorsomedial prefrontal cortex (dmpfc), dorsolateral prefrontal cortex (dlpfc), anterior cingulate (ac), posterior cingulate (pc), inferior parietal lobule (ip), occipital cortex (oc), caudate nucleus (cn), insular cortex (ins), thalamus (th), middle temporal gyrus (mt), ventrolateral prefrontal cortex (vlpfc), frontal operculum (fp), prefrontal/orbitofrontal cortex (pfc/ob), parahippocampal gyrus (ph), nucleus accumbens (na), hypothalamus (hp), amygdala (am), and midbrain (mb).

Family

Interactions among family members influence lifestyle significantly. Types of food purchased and the timing, preparation, size, and composition of meals are all determined by family dynamics as well as leisure-time activities. There is some evidence to suggest that a child's choice of food, behaviour, and physical activity are influenced by their immediate family members. For example, a child's television viewing time can be directly or indirectly related to weight gain. Television advertising can influence food choices. There is possibly increased food consumption while watching television in addition to decreased physical outdoor activity. Weight management programmes that include education of partners (or immediate family) about lifestyle changes, in addition to the overweight subjects themselves, have shown improved outcomes.

Workplace

The workplace is an effective environment to target because of the diverse economic and ethnic population groups seen here. Promoting greater physical activity in a safe environment and increasing the availability of healthy food choices remain the priorities. Some workplaces have even considered incentives for people who are successful in making healthy lifestyle changes. Although these interventions will increase the expenditure for employers and unions in the short term, they will prove cost-effective and beneficial in

2. Dietary changes:
   - Healthy and balanced low-energy-dense diet.
   - Increase intake of fruit, vegetables, and whole grains.
   - Limit intake of high-fat and sweetened foods with high-energy density and low nutritional value.
   - Reduce overall calorie intake by reducing portion sizes and avoid frequent snacking.
3. Increased physical activity (60 minutes/day of at least moderate-intensity physical activity).

the long term by improving the health and productivity of the workforce and reducing sickness and absenteeism.

The following measures could be followed in the workplace:

1. Provision of a safe environment to increase physical activity (e.g. encouraging use of staircases rather than elevators, encouraging use of bicycles, providing open spaces at work for breaks, availability of fitness centres in large workplaces, etc.).
2. Provision of opportunities for organized exercise activities (e.g. yoga, dancing, swimming, group walking, etc.).
3. Arranging educational and motivational programmes on healthy living, weight management, etc. Employees should have access to health behaviour advisors, personal trainers, and nutritional experts, depending on their needs.
4. Increasing the availability of healthy and balanced food choices and limiting the availability of energy-dense foods/snacks such as those provided by vending machines.

Schools

It may take several years or even decades before we can see the benefits of population-based interventions and programmes. One of the most cost-effective and key population groups to target is school children. The positive messages learnt by children about healthy eating and increased physical activity may influence their families and the wider community. Education provided at an early age should be more effective in causing lifestyle changes than in later life. Several countries and healthcare providers have adopted lifestyle intervention programmes targeting schools and educational institutions.

Healthcare network

The identification, prevention, and treatment of overweight and obesity should become part of routine healthcare. General practitioners and community healthcare workers should ensure that there are adequate facilities for measuring weight and they should also offer active support, treatment, and education about obesity and its associated risk factors. Scales for weighing very heavy patients and large size cuffs for measuring blood pressure should be available in all healthcare centres. Recording of height and weight on growth charts for all children and adolescents and the calculation of body mass index for all adults will help identify those at risk and prompt screening of the causes of obesity and associated comorbidities. In countries where healthcare costs are covered by insurance firms, screening

and assessment for overweight and obesity, the availability of lifestyle inventions (5.8) and medical treatments should be considered a priority, as early intervention can lead to substantial savings in the long run by prevention of obesity-related comorbidities and health problems.

Community

Lifestyle intervention programmes are more likely to be effective if they are easily accessible in every local community. Neighbourhood planning is essential to ensure satisfactory distribution of health centres and leisure clubs together with the availability of recreational parks and playgrounds. This is more likely to encourage communities to increase physical activity in a safe environment and engage in a healthier lifestyle.

Regional and national

The role of local, regional, and national policy-makers and planners in the prevention of overweight and obesity and facilitating a safe environment in which to pursue a healthy lifestyle is very profound.

Some important aspects are summarized below, but a detailed discussion about each aspect is beyond the scope of this book.

* Urbanization and its impact on the lifestyle of the population.
* Transport facilities that encourage physical activity in a safe environment.
* Healthcare policies that focus on prevention and education as well as treatment.
* Social security and economic policies that influence dietary and lifestyle choices.
* Media and culture (e.g. advertising regulations).
* Education—targeting key areas such as schools, workplaces, healthcare centres, and social centres.
* Food and nutrition—targeting school diets, supermarkets, local agricultural markets, imported food, regulations on manufacture, packaging, and the advertising of food products.

International and global

Over the last few decades there has been increasing urbanization and movement of populations across countries and regions. Racial and ethnic variations, as well as diverse socio-economic groups, need to be considered during policy-making and healthcare planning (5.9). Globalization of markets and complex restrictions on the importation and distribution of

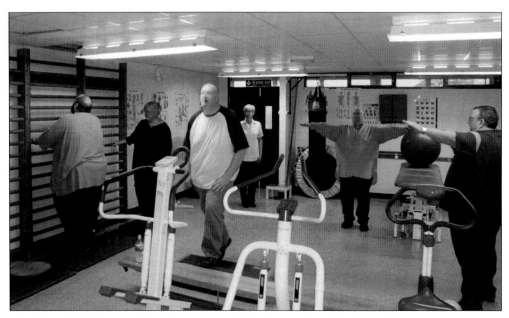

5.8 Exercise programme tailored for high-risk obese subjects who are unable to exercise in routine health centres.

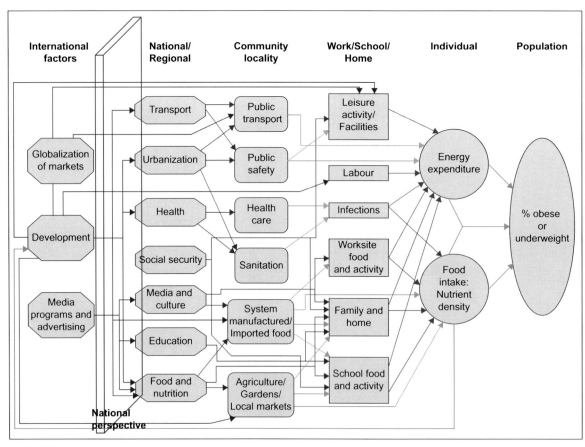

5.9 Social policies and processes influencing the population prevalence of obesity (with permission[7]).

food products and agricultural policies all have a significant impact on lifestyle choices at a population level. Information industry and media advertising (e.g. http://www.nhs.uk/change4life/Pages/Make.aspx) can influence population approaches to a healthy lifestyle (e.g. smoking, alcohol) (**5.9**).

Conclusions: a complex solution to a complex problem

Obesity is the consequence of a complex interplay of a number of factors and variables related to individual biology, dietary habits, and physical activity, and is influenced by genetic, psychological, social, cultural, economic, and environmental determinants. The Foresight Report (the UK Government's programme for tackling obesity and future choices) used a systems mapping approach to capture this complexity and the full obesity system map highlights the fact that a multifaceted approach is needed to tackle the obesity epidemic (**5.10, 5.11**; *see overleaf*).

References

1. Astrup A, Rossner S, Van GL *et al.* Effects of liraglutide in the treatment of obesity: a randomised, double-blind, placebo-controlled study. *Lancet* 2009; **374**: 1606–16.
2. Muhlmann G, Klaus A, Kirchmayr W, *et al.* DaVinci robotic-assisted laparoscopic bariatric surgery: is it justified in a routine setting? *Obes Surg* 2003; **13**: 848–54.
3. Roses AD. Pharmacogenetics in drug discovery and development: a translational perspective. *Nat Rev Drug Discov* 2008; **7**: 807–17.
4. Gautier JF, Del PA, Chen K, *et al.* Effect of satiation on brain activity in obese and lean women. *Obes Res* 2001; **9**: 676–84.
5. Killgore WD, Young AD, Femia LA, *et al.* Cortical and limbic activation during viewing of high- versus low-calorie foods. *Neuroimage* 2003; **19**: 1381–94.
6. Stoeckel LE, Weller RE, Cook EW, III, *et al.* Widespread reward-system activation in obese women in response to pictures of high-calorie foods. *Neuroimage* 2008; **41**: 636–47.
7. Kumanyika SK, Obarzanek E, Stettler N, *et al.* Population-based prevention of obesity: the need for comprehensive promotion of healthful eating, physical activity, and energy balance: a scientific statement from American Heart Association Council on Epidemiology and Prevention, Interdisciplinary Committee for Prevention (formerly the expert panel on population and prevention science). *Circulation* 2008; **118**: 428–64.
8. Kumanyika S, Jeffery RW, Morabia A, Ritenbaugh C, Antipatis VJ; Public Health Approaches to the Prevention of Obesity (PHAPO); Working Group of the International Obesity Task Force (IOTF). Obesity prevention: the case for action. *Int J Obes Relat Metab Disord* 2002; **26**: 425–36.
9. Foresight, Government Office for Science. *Tackling obesities: Future Choices—Project report—Obesity System Map.* London: The Stationery Office, 2007.

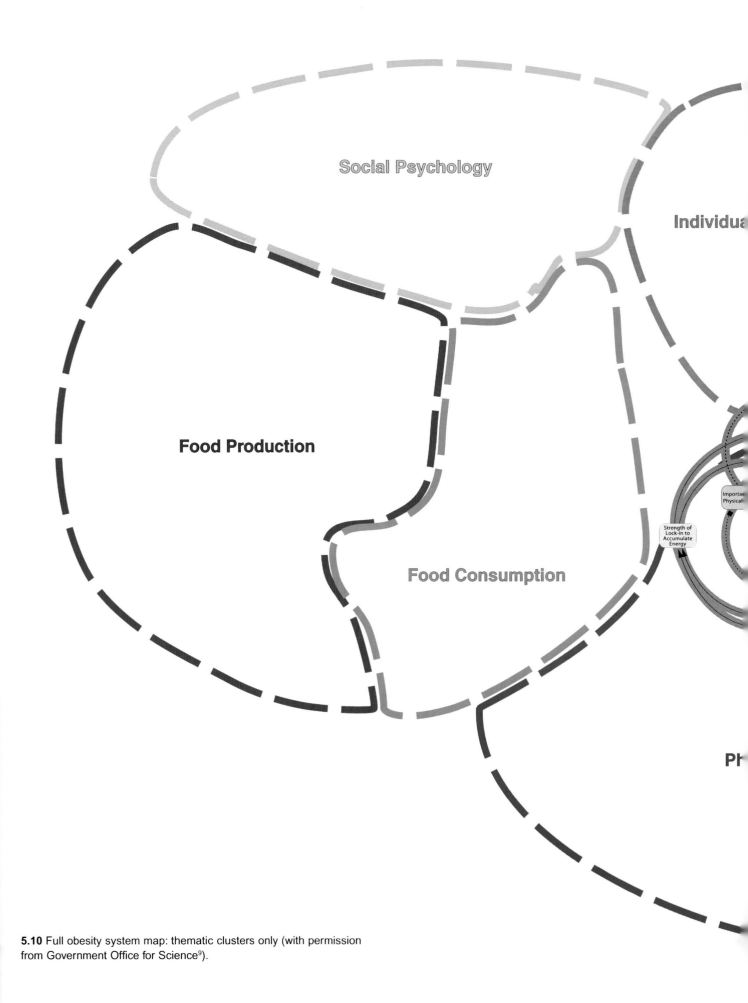

Social Psychology

Individual

Food Production

Strength of
Lock-in to
Accumulate
Energy

Importa
Physical

Food Consumption

Ph

5.10 Full obesity system map: thematic clusters only (with permission
from Government Office for Science[9]).

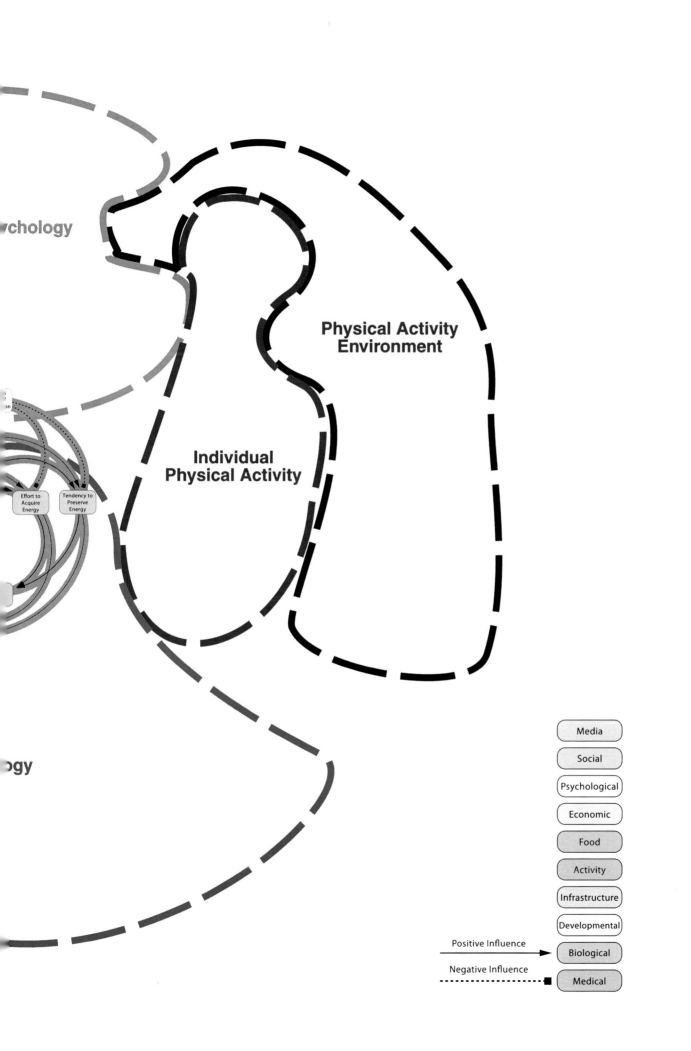

ychology

Physical Activity
Environment

Individual
Physical Activity

Effort to
Acquire
Energy

Tendency to
Preserve
Energy

ogy

Media

Social

Psychological

Economic

Food

Activity

Infrastructure

Developmental

Positive Influence → Biological

Negative Influence ┈┈┈┈┈■ Medical

Full Generic Map
Thematic Clusters (filled)

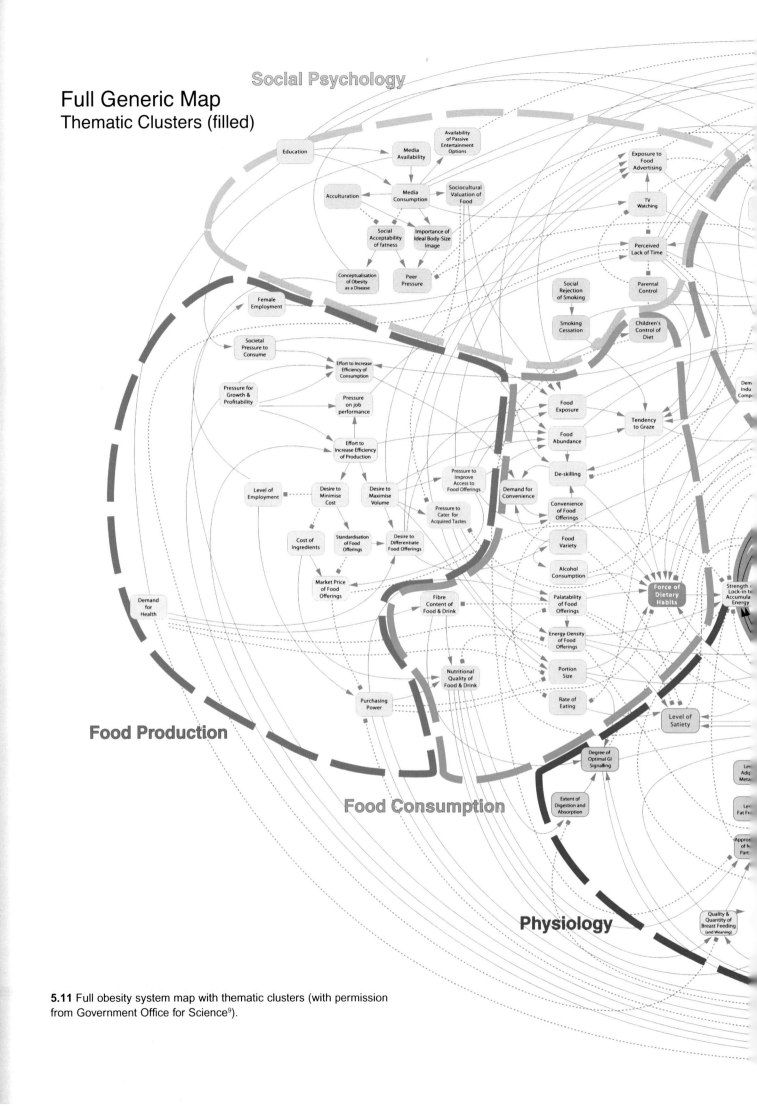

5.11 Full obesity system map with thematic clusters (with permission from Government Office for Science[9]).

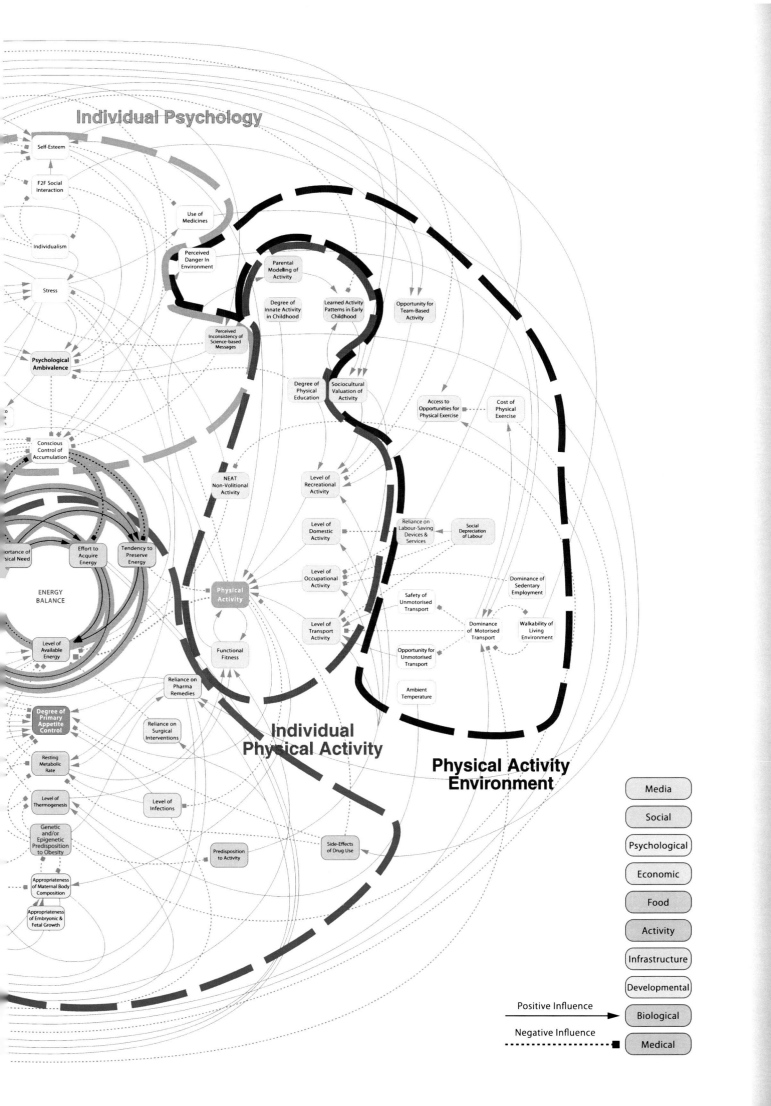

Individual Psychology

Self-Esteem

F2F Social Interaction

Individualism

Stress

Psychological Ambivalence

Conscious Control of Accumulation

...ortance of ...sical Need

Effort to Acquire Energy

Tendency to Preserve Energy

ENERGY BALANCE

Level of Available Energy

Use of Medicines

Perceived Danger in Environment

Perceived Inconsistency of Science-based Messages

NEAT Non-Volitional Activity

Physical Activity

Functional Fitness

Reliance on Pharma Remedies

Degree of Primary Appetite Control

Resting Metabolic Rate

Level of Thermogenesis

Reliance on Surgical Interventions

Level of Infections

Genetic and/or Epigenetic Predisposition to Obesity

Appropriateness of Maternal Body Composition

Appropriateness of Embryonic & Fetal Growth

Parental Modelling of Activity

Degree of Innate Activity in Childhood

Learned Activity Patterns in Early Childhood

Opportunity for Team-Based Activity

Degree of Physical Education

Sociocultural Valuation of Activity

Access to Opportunities for Physical Exercise

Cost of Physical Exercise

Level of Recreational Activity

Level of Domestic Activity

Reliance on Labour-Saving Devices & Services

Social Depreciation of Labour

Level of Occupational Activity

Dominance of Sedentary Employment

Safety of Unmotorised Transport

Dominance of Motorised Transport

Walkability of Living Environment

Level of Transport Activity

Opportunity for Unmotorised Transport

Ambient Temperature

Predisposition to Activity

Side-Effects of Drug Use

Individual Physical Activity

Physical Activity Environment

Media

Social

Psychological

Economic

Food

Activity

Infrastructure

Developmental

Biological

Medical

Positive Influence

Negative Influence

Index